Adam's Rib Disorder

A Misconception of Submission

by

Deborah A. Cosio

authorHOUSE®

AuthorHouse™
1663 Liberty Drive
Bloomington, IN 47403
www.authorhouse.com
Phone: 1-800-839-8640

First published by AuthorHouse 8/13/2009
ISBN: 978-1-4490-0337-1 (sc)
ISBN: 978-1-4490-0338-8 (hc)

Library of Congress Control Number: 2009907800
With permission,
The photographer who did the photo on the cover is Carlos A. A. Pereira,
www.darknesswonder.deviantart.com or e-mail carlp@netcabo.pt.

Art Director of book cover is Lucio Peralta Jr
Email: peralta.one@gmail.com
Website: 3rdcross.com

A couple of the names in this book have been changed out of respect and privacy issues.
The story is true and not embellished. In fact I have toned some situations down
because those details were not necessary in order for me to get the message across.

Graphics on all cover art by Lucio Peralta, peraltaone@yahoo.com

Printed in the United States of America
Bloomington, Indiana

This book is printed on acid-free paper.

FOREWORD

The story you are about to experience will move you to your core. It will cause you to become aware of things that are lying dormant in your soul. I was moved to tears by many of the hardships and frustrations that the author was dealing with. Deborah put into words the complete picture of what many of us women are facing in our day to day life. As for me I had to ask myself, do I suffer from Adam's Rib Disorder? When did the enemy of my soul plant this inner sickness which I had no clue existed?

The author through her words had me experience her grief, pain, shock, and relentless feelings of unworthiness. The unworthiness struck the deepest cord with me because of my childhood situations that left me rooted in self rejection. I was raised by a woman, whom fully lived out Adam's Rib Disorder. She was beaten, and constantly accused of being a cheater for most of her 50 year marriage to my father before my parents received the Lord Jesus Christ as their Savior.

I thank God for the deeper insight that this book has given me. I now live that whole concept of His will in my Life, saying those words, living those words, and meaning those words. Knowing that surrendering my life to God and trusting Him for my healing is the greatest feeling in the world. This is the essence of what Deborah's book made me feel, God is about to move for me, He loves me and I am a King's daughter. Consider doing what Deborah has done by trusting God, and you will see the miracles.

Lydia Suesoff

I would like to dedicate this body of work to my Dad

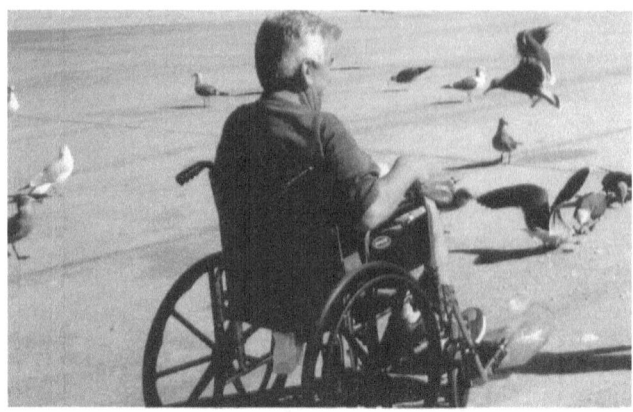

David Ireno Cosio
01/26/1938 * 01/07/2009

I do not think that I will ever get use to not seeing you everyday. Not only were you an incredible father but you also were one of my best friends.

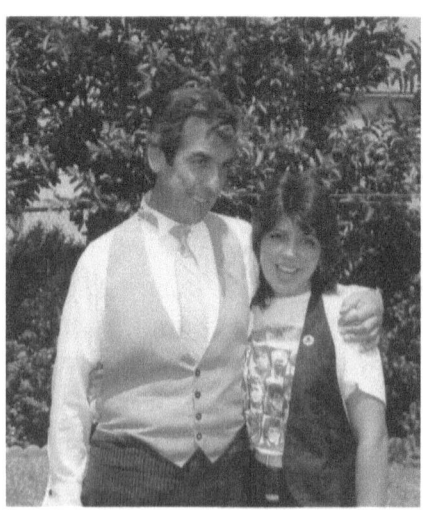

I so enjoyed you and will always remember your great smile and the sound of your laugh. I thank you for always being there, no questions asked. You taught me how to love unconditionally. I know that your last month of life here was drowning in turmoil and strife but know that I have never stopped loving you and look forward to the day that I see you once again in The Kingdom of our Lord.

Acknowledgments

There were so many different people that have truly blessed my family over the past six years. Weather it was helping us through divorce, cancer, the death of my father or in helping me with finishing this book. God blessed me with all of you and I pray that someday I can do the same for you. Until then be blessed and know that I love you all.

I do want to mention two very significant groups who have changed our lives forever. First would be Creative Planet School of the Arts. www.cpsoa.org God brought you into our lives at a time when I was losing grip on my girls, among many other things in my life. You discovered talents in them that I didn't even know existed. In a time when most children would have fallen through the cracks my girls were excelling not only academically but also in every avenue of the arts. I will always remember when I was in chemotherapy treatment for a year and could not afford a penny for tuition. You never even so much as sent me a bill. Know that we truly appreciate you in our lives.

Now to Destiny Community Church International. www.destinycommunitychurch.com Pastor Charley Gallegos, I don't think that I will ever find enough words to describe just how great and significant you are in our lives. God truly brought us to the right place for sanctuary in a time when some people do not even survive. I have come to realize that one of the most important things you have taught me was to stay focused and centered on God while under attack. Through this I have gained my own relationship and faith in God. That is something that will be with me for life. The church as a whole embraced us and loved us through it all. That alone speaks volumes of the leadership at Destiny and I for one, look forward to many more years together.

Table of Contents

1

What Is the Point of Receiving a Gift You Will Never Use?

I believe God has given everybody a special gift. It's a gift that is very specific. Some people have multiple giftings. Understanding that these gifts come from God is of the utmost importance if God is going to be able to utilize these gifts for His Glory and to further His kingdom. I spent fifteen years thinking that I was extremely talented in the arts and in writing, with a flair for expressing myself. I put a lot of time and effort into developing these skills, taking acting classes, voiceover classes, dance classes, and writing classes. I was performing in stage productions as well as dabbling in costume design and even doing choreography. My efforts paid off and I made good progress. Suddenly at twenty-seven, I hit a wall, or should I say a tornado. Within three years, my first marriage of twelve years to Paul, ended due to my choices to sin, and I reaped a divorce. My misery quadrupled by marrying Michael, the man I chose to have the affair with. I unintentionally surrendered my dreams and was in turn put in a position to live someone else's dreams. I allowed myself to be derailed and then completely stifled.

As a submissive wife, that was what Michael expected of me. His dreams were our dreams. It was also how I was brought up. You live what you learn. I don't remember my mother ever expressing a dream or goal of her own; she lived for my dad and us kids. Only my father had dreams, and we supported whatever they were. He was extremely successful, to say the least.

However, God gives each of us a dream, and by my own choice, I gave mine up in the name of what I misinterpreted as love. I spent years trying to suppress my gifts because I was led to believe that there was no need for them. This was extremely hard because my gifts, abilities, and drive were incredibly strong. Whenever I tried to step out, I was quickly slapped back into my place, reprimanded, or quietly sent home with the kids. I cannot tell you how many times Michael and I would be in the middle of an intense argument, and he would say, "This isn't a movie; not everything is a movie, Debbie." This statement was meant to cut the "dramatics."

I could not understand how I could possibly have so many faults. I knew something was wrong, and I was being tolerated, not loved, however, I know now that the dramatics are a part of whom God made me. It was what God deposited inside of me. Not just for my own enjoyment, but so that He could use me as the specific tool that I was made to be. Have you ever tried to use a screwdriver to dig a hole? It doesn't make a whole lot of sense. Yet I ended up spending a lot of my time either trying to be something I wasn't, changing to please others, or hiding who I was in order to be loved. I was also using my gifts for my own desires as well as for those of Michael. It would be nice to blame everyone else for being so off-track but there was no one else to blame but myself. I've learned that people only have the power to throw you off-course if you give them control of your steering wheel. This is what happens when you give man more control over your life than God.

God gave each one of us our own free will. I look back on all my mistakes, and I can't even claim ignorance because God gave me a how-to manual, the Bible, and I would just glance over it once in a while. I look back on my life and I can tell you that every time it felt wrong, it was. The problem was that I was going to force my will through rather than yield my will to the will of God for my life.

One day during a Sunday service, my pastor talked about naming your seed. This meant to write down on the offering envelope what you are believing God for. He said to be specific as to what you are sowing seed for. For the following eight to ten months, I named everything from health to finance on those envelopes. You name it, I wrote it.

Then one day when it seemed nothing was working I threw away my "wish list" and simply wrote "YOUR WILL IN OUR LIVES." For months after, that was all I wrote. Your will in our lives. I figured that Michael and I kept screwing things up and that God was the only one capable of sorting out our completely distorted lives.

As I will go into later, our marriage was a mirage that was actually hiding a whole world of abuses and self-destruction mentally, physically, emotionally, financially, and I'm sure a few others that escape me at the moment. I lived this nightmare for eleven years, and I was desperate to somehow turn it all around. There were a couple of times that I had given our tithing envelope to Michael so that he would see what I had written and be in agreement, but all he said was that it was too vague and handed it back to me. He wasn't into tithing money anyway. He was head of the praise and worship team at church, and he believed that his time and talent was our tithe. That concept never exactly sat right with me. Come to think of it, most of the ways he saw things didn't sit right with me, so I would tithe on my own.

We rarely talked about our future. Our talks were usually him telling me about our future, that is, if he decided to talk to me at all. Most of the time, I would just overhear him telling others about what our dreams were. I would listen to him go on and on about his house that he was going to build.

My opinion or desires were never part of the equation so, if I wasn't going to be included in the decisions of anything from building our home to where to eat dinner, what movie to see, what music we would hear, what T.V. program to watch, where to go on weekend getaways, business directions, or even have a say in money decisions, then I figured, *you know what? I'm going to take this to God.* I was tired of being nothing or being seen as invisible. How could I go wrong? God's will in our lives. What else could you want? Those five words were the most profound words I have ever written. I was about to find out how completely off-track my life had truly become.

Be careful what you ask for. Within six months, my marriage had become completely uprooted. I mean, husband gone, with possible other interests, me still very much in love, and him seeking a divorce. God's will? God's will what? See, the thing is that I had said, "Yes Lord, Your will in our lives! Period!" Not, "Yes Lord, as long as it goes my way.

Or, yes Lord if … I said, "Yes Lord! YOUR WILL IN OUR LIVES!"

I found myself in the middle of a whirlwind, a monsoon that I could not stop. The question was, do I run or do I stand? I was so tired of running. My choice was clear. I had to stand in the middle of this storm no matter how painful or ridiculous I looked or felt. I was experiencing some of the most horrendous things being said to me. It was as if Satan himself was sitting on my chest, and he kept on terrorizing me day and night. I started sleeping with hand towels over my face to soak up the tears so that my pillow wouldn't get wet or the tears flood my ears. I still found myself trying to impose my own will. I knew how to manipulate situations and people's emotions. That is how I had gotten here in the first place, and I wanted no part of it anymore.

The biggest part of accepting God's will is abandoning your own will. I had to accept that they might not be the same. I, for the first time ever, was going to put my life totally in God's care. I found myself in my early forties, on my second marriage, with a fifteen-year-old son, who had already suffered one very nasty divorce, and two young daughters, looking possibly at the same fate. As a Christian, I felt my life looked like a lie. Michael had completely given up on our marriage, so I had to be strong enough to fight for both of us, and to top it all off, I had asked for this. One thing I was sure of was that all of this reeling, gut-wrenching pain was going to birth something positive. I was committed to seeing this through. I wanted to finally succeed in the eyes of God. I was very aware that my life of compromise, or should I say sin, had gotten me here, and it was time for my Christianity to become more than skin deep. I had mastered lip service to God, but now it was going to cost me my heart. God wanted heart service, the real stuff. The funny thing is that I thought I had given God my heart years ago. I don't know how I could have thought that, but I did. I like to compare this awakening to childbirth. You don't fully understand birthing until you go through it and deliver.

For years, I thought that I had devoted my life to Jesus but I was about to find out that I had never taken my relationship with Jesus past acquaintance. God had never become my first husband. Without realizing it, Michael had become my God and he was all too glad to help facilitate this process. I could go weeks without prayer. Yet, my days would be filled with thoughts of "What would make my husband happy?" If I could just keep him happy, then maybe he would love me today. Nine times out of ten, it meant buying him something; I mean, a lot of somethings. When I would get him what he wanted, he was always a little nicer to me. The problem was, it would never last long and I would have to buy him more and more. For instance, I bought him over a dozen registered dogs. I bought bulldogs to boxers, what ever he wanted. Unfortunately he quickly lost interest, and neglect for the dogs set in. I couldn't take care of them. I was supporting the whole household financially by myself and could not work dogs in as well. The health department came and warned me about the excessive dog mess and the smell reported by our neighbors. So rather than deal with it, he just got rid of them.

Buying his love took up a lot of my time. God would get whatever I had left over. My Bible would be for church, that's if Michael decided that we would go. God was never my first or last thought of the day. Furthering His kingdom wasn't even in my vocabulary. I also realized that I had taught my kids the same surface-type Christianity that I had ended up embracing in my life. Divine intervention had begun. OUCH!

2

God Will Get Rid of the Trash; You Have to Clean Out the Can

I pressed in right off the bat. I pressed into God through prayer. I went to my pastors for spiritual guidance. I would listen to worship music to fill and soothe my spirit. I read the Bible and Christian books for ammunition and knowledge. I sought out Godly women for wise counsel, and then, actually, for the first time in my entire life, I embraced the characteristics of Christ. I mean, I embraced and applied them all. I ran from negativity and from the people ready to feed it to me. I was no longer going to hang my head in sorrow and shame, so when I went to church, I looked up during praise and worship. I was seeking God's face. I'm talking a face-to- face experience. I was sorrowful but thankful. I was still unclear of what God's will was, but I knew, for the first time, I was on the right track. This was the worst and best time of my life. I was devastated and excited at the same time. It was time for action, and I had to figure out where to start. As I was taking inventory and surveying what needed to be done, I started with the house. All the rooms looked the same. Huge piles of clutter and trash.

Your physical state as well as the condition of your home tells a lot about what is going on in your life. You couldn't even walk in our rooms, much less our garage, because of the mess and chaos. I started to gut out my house. It was time to get a handle on it all. It's funny because when Michael was home, I used to tell him that I couldn't do it all on my own, that a little help would be nice. He would sit and play video games in eight-hour shifts, but I couldn't get his help with our home or our children. You would be surprised what you can accomplish once you are abandoned by your husband, and once he left, that is exactly what I ended up doing.

With Michael gone, it was also time to deal with the woman in the mirror. She had become someone I couldn't even recognize, and I hated her. That project, however, was a bit much, so I first focused on the house. I had a big truck come on three different occasions and I filled it up with junk that we had accumulated; I trashed it all. I had to keep on going. I would stop a little while to cry but got right back up and kept moving.

One afternoon, I was gutting out the back yard, where there were three tree stumps that I had to remove: two medium ones and one large one. A year before, I had asked Michael to remove these three fruit trees for me because they were too much trouble to keep, and I knew the roots would eventually crack the foundation of our home. The only thing that he managed to do at that time was hack the trees up, leaving about three feet of tree stump on each one, and all the rest was left lying all over the ground, with rotten fruit. I could not even walk out the back door because of the mess, the smell, and the flies. It took my son and I about three or four months of cutting the tops into small enough pieces to be able to gradually throw it all out with the trash. However, the stumps just kept on growing. I kept peeling off the little branches that would pop out, but the foundation was still at risk. I had to gut out the roots, and I knew that I couldn't do it by myself. I had a momentary "Oh my God" breakdown with tears and everything. There was ranting and raving and even some pacing.

Overwhelmed, but not beaten, I found a gardener who was working in my condominium complex and asked if he could help me. I must have looked a sight because he agreed to help without question. He didn't speak English but he could clearly read my distressed face; he called over another gardener and followed me to my yard. If you know anything about tree stumps, it is a very big job. I sat in my kitchen, looking out the window at these two men working on these tree stumps. As I watched quietly, wiping a tear from time to time, I saw them bring five different tools out to work on these roots: a shovel, an ax, a pick, a chainsaw, and a long iron rod with a knife-like end.

They started on the two medium-size ones. They went from one tool to the other. When the chainsaw started smoking, they went to the ax. When they could no longer lift the ax, they went to the rod. Pieces of root landed everywhere. The mess seemed to get bigger and bigger. After about an hour, the first two stumps were out. The men stood and looked at the large one for about ten minutes, as they rested from the first battle. Once they caught their second wind, they were ready. They chopped, hit, cut, and rocked this root back and forth.

After an hour, they left for a break. I went outside to look at the mangled root that would not let go. I could see many roots large and small going in all directions under the concrete. I saw the potential damage. But it wasn't too late. It had not cracked the foundation. As I looked around, pieces of the roots were everywhere. This was much like what had been going on in my life. There were root pieces on the fence, the table, the chairs, the other plants that I had recently planted, and even in the air-conditioning unit. It looked like I was going backwards.

I had to secure the safety of the foundation or it would eventually give out. When the men returned, they had the last root out in about forty-five minutes. This left a huge hole and what looked like a root battlefield or war zone. After I cleaned everything again, it looked awesome. The foundation was solid and the soil ready and rich. It was a reflection of what God was doing in my life. If you tune into God, He will speak to you at every turn, and I understood. I understood my pain. God was in the process of gutting me out. He was getting rid of all roots that threatened my foundation.

We were going back to ground zero. God was getting ready to plant new seed, and He was not going to leave anything that would threaten or kill my God-given destiny. I found that in order to overcome and be victorious, it was not just going to happen. It would have to be intentional and purposed.

3

To Save My Children, I Would Have to Save Myself

Not too long before this happened, I remember praying, "Please God, don't let my daughters become like me. Don't let them follow in my footsteps. Please don't even let them resemble me." I would look at different women and think, "Let them be like her or look like that one or follow this one." I know it sounds sad but it was my reality. And finally God simply said, "In order to save them, you must save yourself. They will follow you. They will follow in your successes as well as your failures. Their future is in your future."

My first thought was, O.K., They did not ask to be born. These are my children. They are my responsibility, and as long as I am breathing, I have no excuse for not leading them with direction and purpose. Therefore, I started walking the walk. That is easy to say, but incredibly hard to do. I just kept putting my trust in God, and I knew that He was at work with all of us. And that is just what happened.

One night I noticed that instead of everyone lying in the living room watching a DVD and eating, we were all in my clean and nice-smelling bedroom. I was lying on my bed reading Tommy Tenney, my seven-year-old was lying next to me reading her children's Bible without help (six months ago, she couldn't even read), and my ten-year-old was on the floor writing out scripture cards, and this was all voluntary.

On New Year's Eve, my kids and I went to an evening church service. My girls generally like to hang out with the kids in the back when there is no "children's church". I went up to the second row and started to press in through praise and worship. A couple of songs into it, my girls both moved up with me, raised their hands, and pressed in with me. During the service, I had one to my left and one to my right. They were taking notes and following with their Bibles. They wanted what they saw me reaching for. I was starting to live something that I wanted to pass on. Spiritually, I was feeding them good fruit instead of junk food. My kids were suffering from spiritual malnutrition as well as suffering from not having a strong mother or father to emulate. I was starting to find myself through Christ, and my girls were loving every minute of it.

I had always thought that life was to be lived to the fullest. I thought that you had to make your mark on this world, and it was up to you to get everything you wanted. Then one day, I saw eternity as the Olympics and life as your training period. Come on! The Olympics! I have never even met an Olympian. If Christianity were your sport, how would you rate? Would you get gold, silver, or bronze or, worse yet, would you just be a spectator? Chances are the way you live life as a Christian here on Earth is a pretty good indication of how you will rate in heaven. You'll go, but what place will you hold? I say, "Realize who you are and go for gold." Life is not just about living. It's about learning, striving, searching, becoming, doing, overcoming, teaching, and embracing everything that God purposed for your life.

An old friend of mine once said, "Why is it so hard for people to do what's right?" It's because we are too busy imposing our own will. Think about it. Look back. Most mistakes you've made, you knew they were wrong but you were willing to deal with the consequences later. I remember making such an astronomical mistake, telling myself that I could wait it out until God moved. Years later, I found out that God would wait me out. Don't ever try to wait out God, because He is definitely better at it. I suggest that you write on your next offering envelope "YOUR WILL IN MY LIFE!" Even Jesus, the Son of God, said, "Thy will be done!" Stop wasting your time. You'll never get it as right as God will. Listen to your head coach and get your training on track. Remember, it's never too late to go for the gold.

If you would have asked me what was first in my life, I would have said, "God." But if you were to examine the evidence, it would have been Michael, which takes me back to the fact that I had made Michael my God. As bad as that sounds, it is more common than you know. I loved my husband more than I loved God. I even loved my kids more than I loved God. In fact, after a thorough investigation, the evidence showed that God missed the top five. I am talking about what got most of my attention and heart. It's easy to say that God is first, but actions speak louder than words. Ask yourself, what is first in your life and then look for the evidence to back it up. What do your actions and words say?

In Matthew 10:37, Jesus said, "Anyone who loves his father or mother more than Me is not worthy of Me; anyone who loves his son or daughter more than Me is not worthy of Me."

When I wrote "YOUR WILL IN OUR LIVES," I gave God the green light to go for it. God will not force His will; instead, He will wait on you to accept His will and then embrace it. I decided to embrace God's will at all cost. In case you didn't know, God will remove from your life whatever it takes to get your complete and undivided attention. My first instinct is to stop this line of thinking because I might offend you, but I would rather take the chance than risk you never knowing. I know it sounds very elementary but look at your life. What evidence do you have that God is most important in your life? Seriously, examine your priorities. What is most important to you? As in any relationship, you will only get out what you put into it. Who is your best friend? How did you become best friends? How much time have you invested in each other?

If the answer to these questions was not God, then how can we say that God is number one in our lives? He is to be your first husband, your first spouse, your first love. This goes for men and women alike. However much you feel for your spouse, God is supposed to mean more; He should be the love of your life. I will be the first to admit that my relationship with God had been dysfunctional as well as conditional, but never again. He now is my first husband, my first love, and I'm going for gold. Don't take it to the extreme, as if I were saying that God is to be your every thought twenty-four hours a day, seven days a week. I'm merely suggesting that God be put in his rightful place. FIRST!

I would also like to say that there are benefits to having God first in your life. It comes with the territory. God having His rightful place will make decisions clearer and easier to make. God being in His rightful place will help you hold sin at bay. You will become more aware of what comes out of your mouth. Soon you will start to take on the characteristics of Christ. You will become a source for God to be able to move through in the lives of others. The list of benefits of Christ in your life goes on and on.

For me, the first results I needed to see were in my children, because they were in a vulnerable state and it was time to step it up on their behalf. It's never too late and most certainly never too early to start fighting on behalf of our seed. I'm talking about our children. If Satan can start on our children from birth, then why can't we? We have been blessed with the honor of being put in charge of our children. On the other side of that coin, we will be held accountable for what they learn as well as for what they don't. Your children will follow what they see on a daily basis. It is one thing to provide the bare necessities for a child, like food, clothing, and a place to sleep, but quite another thing to raise and nurture them, giving them what they need to discover who they are in Christ. It takes great effort to have a vision for them, dream for them, and guide them. If this is not your job, then whose job is it? The world is just swarming with so many bad people out there who are just waiting in the shadows to devour our kids.

If you think I'm sounding dramatic, then I would encourage you to watch the news for one week and tell me how many kids you hear about being beaten or raped or, even worse, killed. Or read up on Samantha Runyon, who was a little girl, abducted from her front yard in a matter of seconds, later to be found dead, having died a horrid death. I'm sure she could tell you a thing or two about what's lurking out there. It is pure evil, and it wants our kids. My problem was that I had jumped into hell head first and then set up house. I got myself in such a horrid position to get so beat up, that I couldn't see through all the blood that my own children were falling further and further away, and the devil was just loving it.

If you don't teach and guide your children through this time of learning and discovery, which we like to call growing up, trust me, they will learn it, but most likely it will be the hard way. With the hard way, which will usually put them on the wrong track, heading in the wrong direction, there is no telling how long it will take them to get their lives back on the right track, going in the right direction.

Look at me. There I was at forty-two years old, asking myself what in the world happened. I was involved in church and "the ministry"; I called myself a Christian, "a true believer." How did I make it so long without deepening my relationship with God? How is it that I thought I had given my life to Him, when I hadn't?

It's because I never put down my own will in order to embrace God's will. I never let my heart become new. I just put a slipcover over my heart to make it look new. I never truly gave God control. I never said, "YOUR WILL IN MY LIFE." I was so confused because I was a conqueror in my humanity. I was young, talented, aggressive, and assertive. I was financially doing great, largely due to my first husband being an excellent provider.

As for my success, my father took me under his wing in business at the age of nineteen and taught me what I needed in order to become an owner as well as a leader. In my ignorance, I took the credit for what I was achieving as my own. I was mistaking my worldly success as me achieving things instead of God, through my dad, working in my life to prepare me for what God had waiting for me. The truth of the matter was I had nothing to do with it other than following my dad's lead. The God in me would rarely get a chance to surface, because "Debbie" would always take matters into her own hands and force it through. Little did I know of the rude awakening that was just around the corner.

4

Never Try to Outwait God.
He is Much Better at It

All God had to do was sit back, watch, and wait me out. The good news, or should I say the awesome news, is that God will wait you out. I had to step out of the little world that I had imprisoned myself in and step into the world that God created. Now, for me, it's a six- or seven-times-a-day thing to say, "YOUR WILL IN MY LIFE." Until it becomes second nature, you will have to fight to abandon your own will. Don't think the devil is going to just kick back and let it happen. You have now become a major threat, so this is where the devil kicks it up a notch or two. He will try anything to get you to take things into your own hands. We have the ability to be an even bigger enemy to ourselves than the devil himself. You would be surprised at how easy we can make life for the devil just in our bad decisions. I had someone ask me, "What is your time limit?" All I could say was, "I don't have one, I will never move in front of God again." Yes, I may be off from time to time, but I will never get behind the wheel again, I have proven to be a terrible driver. I now follow Christ.

Life has actually become a whole new world to me. Just to be aware of things and life around me is a new experience in itself. I now have a respect and love for people and things that before I wouldn't have even noticed. I use to walk low and small but now I am walking tall, with my head up. No, it did not come naturally, because I still felt ugly. But I would hold my head up long enough to notice that my daughter thought nothing of throwing a gum wrapper on the floor or walking past a penny on the floor and not even have a thought to pick it up because its value was so little that it was not worth picking up. I held my head up long enough to see that my sixteen-year-old son thought nothing of spitting on the sidewalk without a care for the person that would have to follow and see it or step in it.

It was time to wake up. I have great, God-given responsibility not just for myself but for the people that God intended me to affect and teach, starting with my own children. The fact that they were so oblivious to their surroundings was just more evidence of my failing in them. I had to wake up in order to wake up my own children.

On Christmas, I took my kids to skid row in downtown Los Angeles to help feed the homeless. As we drove through, I was not prepared to see rows and rows of families, sleeping in cardboard boxes on sidewalks covered with trash. It was so cold that you could see the frost on their breath. This city within a city is an everyday reality. And it exists only twenty minutes away from where we live. We had just come from our home, which was covered with decorations, and had a living room filled with presents. Each one of us had our own bedroom with our own beds and basically our own space in the world. I guarantee that after our visit to skid row, my son thought twice about spitting on a sidewalk that someone may have to sleep on, and that my kids would never simply walk over a penny again.

You must also watch out for the takers in your life. Do yourself a favor and examine the people in your life. Do they add or do they subtract from who you are as a person? If they add to your life and strengthen who you are striving to become, then do not be afraid to embrace them. In fact, you should surround yourself and your family with people of this type of character. If they subtract, then they should have limited access to you. Those who subtract could also be called takers. Takers seek out givers. It's their natural instinct. A taker is also someone who has missed his or her purpose as well. They have not yet found their way back to being on the right track. They usually have no clue that they are even out of position. They feel that to take is their God-given right. Well, let me be the first to tell you that God has no need for designated takers. That is a position that was set up by the devil. That's one of his nifty little seeds, which the devil usually plants when we are children. The parent who is awake and alert is to be the one to weed out all of those bad seeds while a child grows up. As a God-ordained giver, you are to seek out God-ordained receivers.

God will use those whom he has designated as givers to bless receivers. I am a giver, I always have been. The problem that I ran into was that I hadn't given God my heart, so He was unable to guide me in my giving. I would aimlessly give to people. I would squander what God had intended to further his kingdom to further my own life or, even worse, to buy people. An aimless giver with a low self-image is prime territory for a taker. A taker will have a tendency to keep you close at all cost, all the while alienating you from those close to you, and they will take in all areas of your life.

One day, while I was watching a local high school football team win a championship game, it hit me. The giver is like the quarterback. The ball represents the blessing. The quarterback is to find the intended receiver to pass the blessing on to, who will in turn keep moving the blessing in the same direction, this is towards the kingdom. You are supposed to have a common goal, which is to make a touchdown. The quarterback, "the giver," must be specific and direct.

He must also be aware of which receiver is in the best position so that the blessing is not picked off or intercepted by a taker. The quarterback must also be very careful to stay close to those on his team, with the same goal. They will help in protecting him by keeping the takers away, especially since the taker's goal is not the same. In fact, the takers are against us. If given the chance, the taker will try to strip the blessing from the quarterback, and if they can't, then they will try to sack him and try to cause physical or psychological damage. Our goal as givers is to further the kingdom. In order to do that, we must follow God-given direction to find our receivers. If God can give it through you, He will get it to you.

Misguided givers start very young. One day, I noticed that my ten-year-old daughter was collecting loose change around the house. I didn't want to ask her why yet; I wanted to see what her intentions were. I came to find out that she would buy things at school for other kids because she wanted to be liked. She didn't know that that was why she was doing it until we talked about it.

I had done the same thing. I had always done it. Until my forties, it was all I knew. The problem with that is when the money runs out, you are left with nothing because none of it was real. I came to realize I was just as fake as the people and so-called friends that I had bought. When I realized that all I was left with was the person looking back at me in the mirror, all I could do was cry. I really couldn't blame any of those people for leaving. I was investing in takers, and that's exactly what they did: They took from me and then left. On the flip side of that sad story, now that the takers were cleared out, I was about to finally deepen my relationship with God, to get to the next page and finally become a woman of God, in all the fullness and sense of the word.

Finding strength as a woman can only strengthen us as women. In discovering love and respect for who I am as a woman and in finding who I am to God, I found beauty and respect for other women. Before, I was unable to see my value, and in turn, I could not see the value of other women. My perception was to compete with other women. I wanted to hold them at bay so that they could not hurt or take from me. Well, yes, that is just another one of those nasty little seeds that the devil planted in me at an early age. I would keep my blessings at bay because I always kept women at arm's distance. God has blessed us with the ability to bring forth life through our own bodies. Yet, we bring forth so much pain and death with our mouths and our actions. We have the ability to give life to our children as well as our husbands, yet divorce and broken families are so common. What are we doing wrong? The Bible says, "They will know we are Christians by our love." I suggest that we had better figure out what we are doing wrong. We should start loving one another because I am personally tired of pain and death and I long for joy and life.

5

... And the Blind Shall See

One of the greatest gifts I have ever received from God was the ability to hear His voice. We have a tendency to call it woman's intuition but in actuality that still, small voice is God whispering right into your ear. Or when you might say, "I don't know, I just have this feeling," that is God quickening your spirit. If you tuned into God, you would be amazed at how often God will speak to you. I knew that Michael was about to go to the point of no return. I knew that he was toying with the idea of an affair. I fought like crazy to keep him from taking that fatal step, but he was already determined on seeing it through. I remember him sitting in the kitchen trying to come clean with me. He said, "I opened my heart to another woman." I locked into a mode of desperation. The day before he left, I begged him to stay with us. I literally begged him to hold me or even kiss me, and he simply couldn't. He couldn't even look me in the eye. Now that is what I call a serious blow to a woman's psyche.

Even after he left the house, I was in prayer. As long as I did not know for a fact that he was having an affair, then I could keep fighting. I would call him on his cell phone to pray with him over the phone, and he would just say, "I don't think you're supposed to call me and do that, I think you're supposed to pray for me on your own." How could I have been so stupid to believe in this guy, when everyone else could see him for who he really was?

When two months had passed, my marriage was quickly fading. I started looking for my photo album with pictures of our wedding to give myself something to focus on. I looked and looked and looked but could not find it anywhere. In the blink of an eye, another five months came and went, and I was still looking for the photo album. By then, my appearance was really starting to suffer. I looked like death warmed over with swollen eyes and dark circles. I was just lost in my sorrow, heartbreak, and embarrassment of being discarded like garbage, as well as being so publicly wronged. I had put everything on my relationship with Michael and I lost it. That is what happens when you put everything on man and not on God.

Then one morning, the Lord told me, "Today is the day," and I thought to myself, "For what?" And He said, "You know."

And you want to know something? I did know. I knew that I had loved blindly. I refused to see Michael for who he really was. I thought that I could love enough for both of us. So all day, I had nervous knots. What was God going to show me? I dropped off the kids at school, went to work, went to Curves, picked up my son from school, went to the market, and still nothing, but I knew it was coming. I called Michael, I was very emotional, and I told him that God wanted me to see him for who he really was, that I had loved him blindly and God said no more. I was to realize all that he had done to me and to stop making excuses for him; I was to stop.

Michael's response was so predictable: "What about what you did to me?" I wasn't going to get anywhere with him, and I knew it.

I went on to make dinner, pick the girls up from school, feed them in the car on the way to rehearsal for a play we were doing at church, and then tried to direct the play. At about 8:30 p.m., there was an accident during rehearsal; Tiffany, my younger daughter, hit her head pretty badly, and I rushed her to the emergency room at a nearby hospital. After the first two hours of just waiting, a family friend took my other two children home and I stayed with Tiffany alone. For the next three hours, we sat in emergency, holding ice on Tiffany's head.

As it turned out, she was fine; her injury was not that serious, and she was released. On our way home at about 12:30 in the morning, it was a quiet drive with my little girl curled up in the front seat, sound asleep. I felt a quiet peace as I sat back and exhaled very deeply with a sigh of relief because I had made it through one more day. I was going to turn the radio on when all of a sudden I heard the voice of God say,

"Are you ready?"

And I thought to myself, "NOW????? I went all day without so much as a peep out of you, and now at 12:30 in the morning, you ask me now?" Instantly, the nervous knots were back in my stomach. I took a moment to think and then I simply said, "YES, of course!! Why not? Yes now. What?" Then He said, "Go to HER house." And I thought, "What?!!!" It had been seven months, and I had never gone to the home of the suspected "other woman," who, by the way, just happened to live in the same condominium complex as we did. I would always tell myself that I had more self-respect than that. Besides, Michael had always denied being with her or that he was seeing her, so why would I? It just seemed pointless. But God said, "Because now you're ready."

As I drove my car towards her driveway, my headlights slowly revealed his car, which he obviously tried to hide up on the grass on the side of her condominium beyond the driveway. I instantaneously froze while my hands gripped the steering wheel. I could actually feel my heart pounding while the tears began streaming down my face. I found it hard to breathe and was actually having physical pain in my heart area. I started to mutter out loud, "No, God … NOOOO!! That's not his car, that can't be his car, it's not." I heard the voice of God saying, "I need you to see him for who he is; I can no longer allow you to live in darkness. This is not what I wanted for you."

Even after hearing that straight out of the mouth of God, I was still saying out loud, "No, no, no, it's not his car." I looked at my little girl, curled up asleep in the front seat, and then looked at the dark house with no lights on and said, "No, this is a mistake, he is not capable of this." For thirteen years, I had poured everything I was and everything I had into this guy. This was not happening to me after all my pain and suffering. I opened my car door and found myself walking towards his car to touch it. Somehow, I thought to myself that maybe this was just a nightmare, and if I reached out to touch it, that it would just somehow disappear. Everything felt like I was in slow motion as I walked towards his car. I reached out with my hand all the while saying, "No! That's not his car!" My hand slowly came to rest on the cold hood of his car, then the other hand, and then I slowly bowed my head in defeat while watching my tears hit the hood of his car, making perfect little circles that glistened in the moonlight.

I heard the voice of God again; this time, He said, "From this day forth, you are healed of your blindness. This is who he is, this is what he is, I never asked you to love blindly, this was your will, not mine. I have so much more for you but I cannot give it to you until you let go of this." Just then, I threw my head back, and the movement of my long hair caused a motion sensor light to go on.

At first, I thought it was the porch light and that he was coming out. I looked back at my car with my little girl still asleep in the front seat, and I ran, jumped into my car, and drove away as quickly as I could. All I could do was scream, "O.K., O.K., O.K., I get it! I see it, ALL RIIIIIGHT!!! No more, please no more." I felt as though I was going to vomit. The tears would not stop, it was as if they had a mind of their own. I was frantic to the point of panting like a dog. Now I knew that the fight was on. Not a fight between my husband and me, but the fight between my flesh that wanted to act out and my spirit that wanted to get a grip on what God wanted to deposit into my soul.

I found myself wondering, who in the world do I reach out to? Do I call someone who will jump in a car with me and go cause some damage (because I knew the right girl for the job), or do I call someone who will speak truth and wisdom to me and keep me in my house with my kids? I pulled up to the house and got my daughter upstairs and into bed. When I came downstairs, I was literally pacing back and forth from my living room to the kitchen and back again. I would put my hand on the doorknob to leave and confront them both, and then I would let go of the door and pace some more. I would fall onto the couch crying and then stand, determined to take a stand against this injustice. If there had been someone with me that night in my living room, I often wonder if they would have seen two of me because that is how real the fight was between my flesh and my spirit.

I called his cell phone and left a message to the effect of "All this time, you have been trying to make all your family and so-called friends believe you were trying to right a wrong of our relationship because we started in adultery and because you had come to realize that you were never really in love with me, and all this time it was really about another woman."

For the past seven months, I had been embracing the things of Christ, now it was time to use the characteristics of Christ for battle. I had learned to do the God thing. I fell to my knees and just cried out to God, "Help me, Lord, Lord, Lord, please help me move in your will." I rolled over onto my back and stared at all the pictures on my walls, trying to hold onto reality and refuse insanity. I decided to call my mother-in-law. Actually, God screamed at me to call my mother-in-law.

Within ten minutes, my husband was pounding at my door, screaming obscenities. You have to understand that God will always give you what you need; you just have to ask. I thank God that I called my mother-in-law and had her on the phone, because I believe that she was the only reason he left without incident. Knowing that she was on the phone, listening to him make a fool of himself, was the main reason, I believe, he stopped pounding.

After about five minutes, he simply bowed his head, looked at me through the window, reached out his hand, and whispered, "I'm so sorry." Then, as if in defeat, realizing there was no way to undo what had been done, he just walked away.

That night had such a devastating potential for violence, the police and my kids witnessing it all, and I just could not let that happen. I had to take the right road on this. For the first time in my life, I was equipped to fight the way God wanted me to battle because I was prayed up, praised up, worshiped up, counseled up, and read up, and I had my spiritual armor head to toe and then some. Winning the battle doesn't mean getting your way, it means God's will coming forth and you carrying yourself as a Christian, which means Christ-like. It's easy to be Christ-like when everything is all good. Try it when it feels as if your whole world is coming to an end or when you have been as defiled, as I felt that night. Try it when you feel gutted like a fish.

I spent four hours face down on the ground, in the dark, in my room that night, but by the time I fell asleep, at 4:30 in the morning, I had prayed for them both. Not that they would live happily ever after (please, I hadn't made that much progress), but that the Lord would have His way in their lives and that He would keep me from escalating the situation. It was obvious that my husband had made his decision and I, in turn, had made mine. I walked away as God had instructed me; that is what I call winning the battle.

Don't get me wrong, it was a horrible, horrendous, and excruciating night but worth every minute because I had made it to the next level with flying colors. After twelve years, Michael's hold and control over my life, heart, mind, and spirit was broken. I experienced a rebirthing, if you will. There is a reason a baby comes out screaming and kicking, but once the baby realizes it is going to be O.K., it can fall asleep and so starts its trust. Once I realized I was a bit battered but going to live, I started a new trust in God and just fell asleep in His arms.

6

A Picture Can Say a Thousand Words

This brings me back to the photo album. About two weeks after this horrid yet glorious realization and awakening, I finally came across the photo album I had been looking for over seven months. I opened a closet, and there on the top shelf, I saw a corner of it. As I reached for it, God told me, "I have something I want to show you."

I thought, "Oh Lord, am I up for this one?" I went to the kitchen and sat down, put my feet up, and opened the album. I was gripped with a flood of emotions, and not too many of them were on the good side; in fact, not one of the emotions was pleasant. This was definitely not what I was expecting. I was looking at pages and pages of a beautiful, sexy, attractive, vibrant, adventurous, talented, life-giving woman who no longer existed. I wondered why it was that she never knew she was all of those things. Why? Married twice, for twelve years each time, and she never knew? I was pulling out picture after picture as my tears were hitting them. I stared in amazement. I felt as though I were mourning someone who had died. To top it off, I had done nothing to help her. In fact, I just sat back and watched it happen. She was so beautiful and had such potential, joy, and hope, and now she was dead. What a wasted life, I thought. She had spent her life pouring into others, into their hopes, into their dreams, all with the hopes of just being loved, and it just never happened.

I ended up putting the pictures into an envelope and carrying them around with me for days. I must have looked at them at least three times a day, then I would look in the mirror and I would think to myself, "I can't blame them for not loving me," because I could not see myself as lovable. Then in a moment of clarity, I thought, what if the woman I now see in the mirror still possesses the things that the woman in the pictures possessed? I can guarantee, like the woman in the pictures, the woman in the mirror does not see anything that remotely resembles beauty or being attractive, sexy, vibrant, adventurous, or talented, much less life-giving. So now, I am left to figure out what has gone wrong. Why do I have this ugly duckling syndrome? Why have I settled for so little? Why do I have no self-worth? Why can't I see who I truly am? When did all this mess get started?

Satan started planting negative seeds in my spirit a long time ago. When I was five years old, my mother discovered that her grandfather was molesting me right in the midst of my family. He would sit me on his lap and cover the both of us with a blanket and proceed to fondle me. Once my mother figured out what was going on, I never saw him again. I believe that this is where my self-worth started to come under attack.

Then when I was ten years old, I was abducted and sexually violated by a familiar man in the neighborhood. He was teaching kids in the area how to ride horses. He "groomed" me for about a month by making his touch a familiar occurrence. Then one day, he took me for a long drive in his car and molested me. It was extremely confusing because the act was mixed with good sensations, which sounds sick but true. As a child, I was not prepared to process this but my spirit knew I had been violated.

My mom found me crying, and I told her and the police exactly what happened but the man, when questioned, said that he was just removing thorns from my underwear. As I got older, I figured that I had not been affected as badly as one might expect, maybe because the ordeal was not a violent one. This would prove to be the continuation of a series of unfortunate events.

Now my spirit was growing worthlessness alongside broken trust. Those seeds were never pulled out of my spirit and later would grow out of control. I had made it through all of high school without being asked out on a single date. Not one dance, football game, or school function.

I had met Paul, my first husband, through church when I was fifteen years old, and I was in love right off the bat. I knew that I was not his cup of tea; in fact, Paul had it bad for a girl named Sandra. It was obvious that I had a major crush on him, and he would always try to be gentle about not hurting my feelings, because he did not feel the same for me. During the three years that I was waiting on God to show Paul that I was his answer to life and should become his wife, I experienced three different guys through church, and in all three cases, I was the other girl and I always lost out to the main squeeze. So the not-being-good-enough seeds that had grown into weeds with thorns was now out-of-control bushes, covered with sharp, pointy thorns. Needless to say, I had sustained a lot of damage by the time I was able to force my will of being a wife on husband number one.

My persistence wore Paul down, and three years later, he took me out on our first date, which was grad night at Disneyland.

It was on June 13, 1979; the fact that I know that date right off the top of my head tells how obsessed I was. I felt lucky that this great guy would even go out with me. A year and a half later, we would marry. Looking back, I realized something: In our twelve years of marriage, he never once looked at me the way he would look at Sandra. Never! And I accepted that.

I loved everything about this guy; he was talented, funny, and clever, and he had eyes to die for. However, the pain he caused me, though not intentionally, proved to be emotionally fatal. I believe he tried to love me but it just never came. I never became necessary in his world. He was a police officer and worked up to 80 hours a week. So in order to deal with our new life together, alone, I chose to fill the void with whatever I could. I started drinking, which increased my desire to smoke. I was nightclubbing a lot and went to every concert that came to Los Angeles. I threw myself into acting, and I loved going dancing. On holidays, he went with his family and I went with mine. As long as I didn't pressure him, he was cool with it. We led completely separate lives, but hey, I still had my man, or so it seemed.

After eight years, I knew it was time for me to have a baby; I said ME and not us. The ME, ME, ME part and not US is one of those little side effects to living together, separately. The concept was very big in the eighties, which might explain the massive divorce rate in the nineties. I kept telling my husband I was ready to be a mother, and yet I could not figure out why he kept side-stepping the issue.

Then one day, he just simply sat me down and said, "I don't think I can be married to you for life." Well, you could have knocked me down with a feather; I was devastated. I think we can say that the seeds of not being good enough were now a full-blown forest. This was the first real pain of heartbreak I had ever felt. This blow was to my soul. The possibility of us not making it till death do us part had never even entered my mind. What was I supposed to do with that? I mean, I was one of the least demanding women I knew. He was able to pursue any and all of his dreams, from police work, writing, and cartooning to running marathons, anything. I never got in his way, I never said no. I loved that he had a passion for his work and his writing. How could I ever try to take that from him when it was what he loved? Did you get that? It was what "he loved." I had given him all of me yet once again, I was not good enough. In all fairness, allow me to reword that: I was not the love of his life.

Nevertheless, he was still my best friend, and I wanted to have a baby. I had a pretty good feeling that we were not going to make it but I still wanted a child. A year later, we had Eric. The one thing I think we would both agree on was that Eric was and is still the best thing we ever did together.

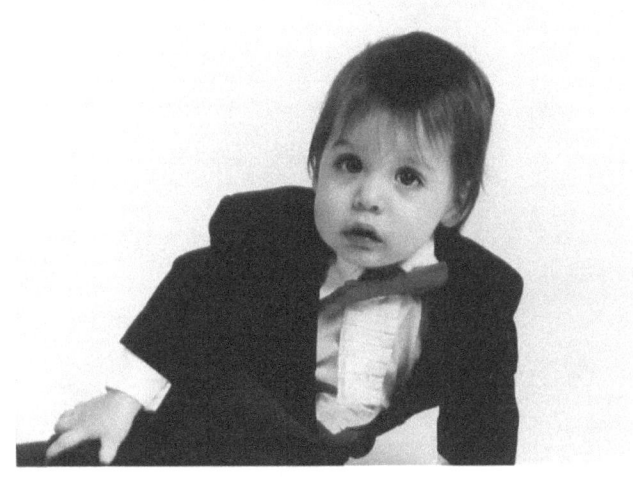

Eric Paul

We still stayed together another four years but we never sought out help to make our marriage work, and without help, I think the bottom line was that I just could not recover from that initial blow of him saying, "I don't think I can be married to you for life." I was not necessary in his life, so I made him unnecessary in mine. Still, he never fell in love with me, and the worst was yet to come.

7

You First Must Be Complete Within Yourself

Perhaps in the eyes of the world, I was a smart, successful businessperson, running my father's very successful sheet metal company as the owner. Over a million dollars a year would pass through my hands. I was aggressive, confident, bold, and beautiful. However, as a woman, in all her beauty, I was looking for approval through the eye of a man, and I could never achieve it; I only suffered losses. I never had experienced a good or friendly ending. In all my relationships, I was made to feel as if I fell short. I should have been at the top of my game, and yet I was in the gutter.

I was desperate to find anyone, or should I say any man, who would find value in me. Without someone to love me, I felt that I was not complete or whole. I seemed to always be rejected in one way or another. This is a very, very bad place to find yourself.

I was not a streetwise woman, and now I was out in the world alone because, remember, I had made my husband unnecessary so I was living life as "I am woman, hear me roar," all the while I was without the covering of my husband. Let me just say that it did not take long for me to be devoured. Maybe, if I had just taken a moment to let the smoke clear, maybe I would have given God a chance to step in and take over our lives. Unfortunately, my world was about to really take a turn for the worse.

It took me a year and a half to get my divorce, and three days later,

I married for the second time. This time, I would mistake someone wanting to possess me for someone wanting to love me. This is where the blindness thing crept in, because I wanted to be wanted at any cost. In my second marriage, I endured mental abuse, verbal abuse, financial abuse, and yes, physical abuse, all this before I even said, "I do."

The following is an actual journal entry from two years before my second marriage. It was when I considered this guy to be a friend.

> **For the last week he has, for some reason found it necessary to put me down every chance he gets. Whether it be my son, my house, my opinion, my marriage, my looks, body, taste, driving, or anything that has to do with me. He completely crushes me from the inside out. I thought he was a true friend. Actually, at one point I know he was. Now he finds pleasure in ripping at me and it gets more severe when his partner is around. At this point, there is not anyone who makes me feel worse than he does. He reduces me to tears all the time, I just can't tell him.**

So how is it possible that two years later, I would actually marry this person? One time, he sat on my chest and choked me with both of his hands around my neck until my lips turned blue. You often hear battered women tell their story and you ask yourself, "Why in the world do they stay?" I can only speak for myself, when I say that I was desperate to be loved.

I was not an ignorant woman, just a misguided giver. I was intercepted on the way to my destiny. I had allowed this guy to come into my life, marriage, and home, and ultimately he consumed me. When someone consumes everything that you are, it makes you feel needed or necessary, which is what I had looked for my whole life. I mistook the intensity of the violence or the intensity of control for intensity of love. You do not know that eventually, you will die; you cannot see that it is anything but love.

Here is another journal entry from two years into my second marriage.

> **Last night we had a party. He never came near me to hug, kiss, or even touch. The whole night I watched him from afar. He was so happy laughing and smiling from ear to ear. His laughter**

sounded so heavenly because he does not have much laughter in his life. I was dying because I was not a part of it. However, I am glad it is a place he can still find. I want to learn to at least find pleasure in him from afar. If I can see him smile, I will settle for that. You know something, his smile is so beautiful. If I could just have one smile a day, I will make that all I need.

Year after year, I wrote pages of the same stuff. Here is three years into my second marriage.

Whenever you're away from me, An emptiness consumes me
I start to wither from within, Like a flower without water
If you do not come back soon, I will dry up and only resemble
what you once made me
I lie in bed and close my eyes, and try to hear you breathe
I turn to see your silhouette; I know that I am alone
My life is at a stand still every time you leave
I wonder if another is hanging on your sleeve
Don't ever let me leave your heart, I know there could be many
A dime a dozen some would say and I am just a penny

I am including parts of my journal so that you can see how truly blind I was and how little I was made to feel. Some might say that I was just plain stupid. Trust me when I say that it's not that simple; I have given this a lot of thought and I really believed that God would turn it around, which is bizarre because this relationship was not His idea in the first place. Now, looking back, I realize that here is where I completely abandoned myself.

JOURNAL ENTRY 11-1-93
Do not kid yourself any longer. You are not and never have been...
An actor
     A director
     A producer
     A writer
     A businesswoman
     A leader

> A counselor
> INTELLECTUAL
> INSIGHTFUL
> Or a speaker

It seems like I spend all of my time trying to prove I'm one thing or another. But you know maybe if I was what I've always thought I was, then I would be, instead of always fighting to prove that I am.

I am not ...

> A choreographer
>> A dancer
>> Or a costume designer

Not only am I not, but I don't even need any of these titles to be what I really am.

> 1st A wife
> 2nd A mother

And   3rd A housewife

That's it. That's all. No more or less. From here on out I have no views or opinions on things I am not qualified on.

I am where I am going. It's seems as though I've been waiting for my true purpose to be revealed. I am nothing more than what I am. There is no big, mysterious purpose. I am not a career woman. I'm not a woman of great intuition. I will no longer speak on what I'm not, just on what I am. I am not a woman of great taste. I am not a person of the Theatre. I saw maybe twenty plays on Broadway, which does not mean I know good theatre. I am not a woman of diamonds and $100 perfumes. I am not a woman of class. I cannot read people. I haven't read a book from beginning to end in all of my life. I have to come to grips with all of this. I've been fooled for far too long.

I am not qualified to give people advice. I can't even help my own husband because he says that I'm too busy and lost trying to be everything I'm not. He has to go to other people for understanding. He is on the phone right now, behind closed doors, confiding in someone else. He says he has to because I know nothing about what he's going through.

Michael's whole point was to make me feel like garbage, and he succeeded. God had nothing to do with any of this. I knew where I had screwed up in my first marriage; living separate lives did not work before, and I did not want to make the same mistakes again. I thought that I could fix this. Except that what would happen is that Michael would live his life and my son, our two daughters, and I would only be allowed to watch him live his life. He was an evangelist, supposedly, and would always speak of his awesome wife but would rarely introduce me. He never would wear his wedding ring because he said rings bothered him. As a Christian rapper and singer, he preferred that the girls and I stay home while he was performing so that we would not distract him while he was "ministering." He said that it was his work and that he needed to be focused. He would also require that I have no life, he said that if I went anywhere while he was "ministering," that he would not be able to concentrate. I did not want to add any pressure on him so the kids and I always stayed home.

8

How Much Can One Woman Take?

I would accept whatever crumbs Michael would decide to throw my way. I had gotten marriage all wrong again.

In Genesis 2:23-24 it reads: The man said: "This is now bone of my bones And flesh of my flesh; She shall be called woman, for she was taken out of man." For this reason a man will leave his father and mother and be united to his wife, and they will become one flesh.

The two will become one, not together but separate and certainly not both living for one. I was living for Michael and he was living for himself. My life was completely out of balance once again. I was making bad choices but was willing to pay the price because I felt like I was needed and loved.

I thought Michael was in love with me, and that made all the pain worth it. I became an expert at covering up for him. I wore whatever hid the bruises, and if by chance someone did see them, I came up with a story on the spot. I remember running into one of his sister's friends at the market, and I had a big, USDA choice kind of bruise on my arm from being pushed into a wall. I came up with, oh I fell over some toys.

I remember walking away, thinking, I know she knows, no one could be that clumsy, but hey, at least he wanted me, at least he loved me. I tried to model myself as the wife the Bible speaks of. I was submissive, supportive, nurturing, self-sacrificing, understanding, and protective. Michael was eight and a half years younger than I was, and I told myself that I would be able to hold on until he grew up. The problem was that his behavior had nothing to do with immaturity. It had everything to do with lack of character and I had fallen for this guy hook, line and sinker. Meanwhile, Michael wanted a son, a son who would carry on his name. We had tried twice and we had two daughters, two of the most beautiful, talented, and joyful girls you could ever meet, but this just wasn't good enough for him.

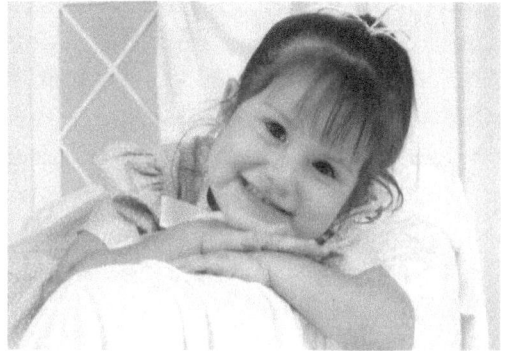

Cheyenne

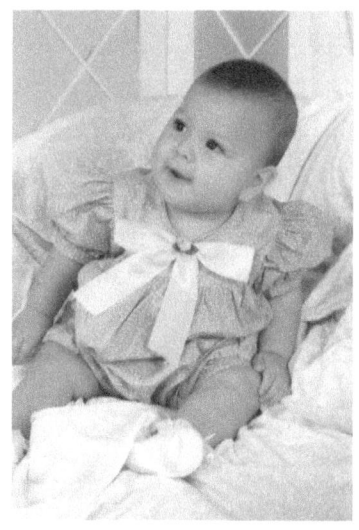

Tiffany

I was already thirty-six years old and was basically a single mother of three as it was, because he was living his own life and we were only allowed to watch. Even though the marriage was in a shambles, he still wanted to keep trying to have a son, because he said that my son would never really be his own.

I saw that there was very little involvement in our girls' lives as it was, and if we had a son, it would only make it worse for them. He knew that I did not want to try again but he kept trying to get me pregnant, so I decided to have my tubes tied even though I knew that this would further lessen my position in his life, but I knew that if I ended up alone, I could still handle three kids by myself.

Michael finally left me after twelve years of marriage, telling me that he never was in love with me. He said he was trying to make things right again because he felt as if he had broken up my first marriage. I would like to set the record straight. First, my first marriage was over with or without Michael, because we never sought help. When I left my first husband Paul, it was not with the intention of getting with Michael. In fact, I would have bet the farm against that union.

Second, Michael never had that much moral fiber. I had set myself up for this; I provided everything for him. From his car, his gas, his clothes to his food and his spending money, his toothpaste, toilet paper, even the roof over his head, I supplied it all. He didn't even have a job; he'd made a choice of convenience, by finding someone who would take care of him, and he knew if he left me, he would also lose all the conveniences, from my car that he drove to the roof over his head.

I would sometimes have to leave work at lunch because he would call and wanted me to bring him food. He was a taker and a master at manipulation with a black belt in selfishness. The physical abuse subsided a couple of years into the marriage but the mind games and belittling would prove to have a far greater effect because I could no longer see myself as anything of value. If I sat next to him and put my hand on his leg, he would ask me not to touch him.

One time he was playing basketball outside in the front yard with a young girl from across the street, and I felt uncomfortable or jealous so I went out there and sat down to watch. Love would have said, "Hey babe, you wanna watch?" But no, Michael said, "What in the hell are you doing out here? Go inside," so I did; I sat on the couch and turned the T.V. on, all the while tears were just streaming down my face. And of course, the experience would not be complete without him coming in later on and making me feel like a possessive wife who made it hard for him to breathe.

Everything was always all about him. It seemed like he was mean and cruel to me because that was his way of making me pay for him not loving me. In private, his pet name for me was Baby Huey, and he insisted that that big, fat, dopey duck was cute. I have yet to find a woman who would appreciate that kind of compliment. He had a sick gift for putting me down and trying to disguise it as a nice thing to say.

Thinking back, I realize that Michael disliked most things about me, from my music to my toes. How do I know this? He would tell me all the time, from the way that I spoke and the words I used to the sports teams I liked. If I liked it, it was stupid. I can recall one time when I wanted to watch my favorite football team on T.V., and he told me that I was not allowed to watch them in his house, so I didn't. I just never could seem to make him happy. I would drive to three different places to get the foods he liked but when I got home and served him there was always something that I missed or forgot.

I gave myself over to abuse by my own choice, in exchange for what I thought or perceived as being wanted and loved. But deep down in my heart, I knew the truth. I think everyone did. I sometimes ask myself, "Why didn't anybody step in and help me?" But there is nothing anyone can do to save you from abuse unless you want to be saved. Looking back, I did have a few friends that did try to talk to me about the illness of our situation, but they were quietly dismissed, without discussion, never to be called again. I allowed Michael to isolate me completely. I protected him at all cost. There was only one person who I always went to for help, and she was related to him. I figured that whatever I told her, she would still love him because if I had gone to anyone in my circle of family or friends, they would have helped me get out and also put him in jail. Unfortunately, the person I picked to go to just ended up helping me to sustain this hell of an existence for years because it was what she knew. That's as bad as a drug addict going to another drug addict to kick drugs. It's not going to happen; they can only help you maintain and survive. I had become an expert in hiding and concealing. It was apparent that I could no longer hide the fact that something was terribly wrong; I could only hide the seriousness and extent of the abuse I was incurring. Please get me the instructions for this thing called life.

1 Corinthians 13:4-8: Love is patient, love is kind. It does not envy, it does not boast, it is not proud. It is not rude, it is not self-seeking, it is not easily angered, it keeps no record of wrongs. Love does not delight in evil but rejoices with the truth. It always protects, always trust, always hopes, always preserves. Love never fails.

I had often heard preachers refer to the Bible as our owner's manual, which would mean that we are supposed to first read it and then apply it to our lives. If I had read this and compared this passage to my second marriage, there would be no way I would have been able to explain or defend my decision to marry that man only three days after my divorce was final. It was the wrong decision on so many levels, not just for me but for everyone involved. My desire to be wanted or loved took precedence over everything else, and perhaps that is why my decision to marry again was never thought out. I knew the answer would be to run the other way, and I was not willing to accept it. I was going to make this relationship work, and in the process, it cost me myself. I am finding that many women make this mistake. We just do not wait on God. God NEVER intended us to be abused in any way, shape, or form. We choose to accept abuse because we have lost sight of our value. Let's read the scripture again:

1 Corinthians 13:4-8: Love is patient, love is kind. It does not envy, it does not boast, it is not proud. It is not rude, it is not self-seeking, it is not easily angered, it keeps no record of wrongs. Love does not delight in evil but rejoices with the truth. It always protects, always trust, always hopes, always preserves. Love never fails.

It cannot be said any clearer than that: Love never fails; we do. I don't know what tomorrow will bring or even what the next hour will bring, for that matter. However, I now choose to wait on God, no matter how long it takes or what it involves, it has to be God.

I have become the kind of Christian that the devil has to worry about. I recently heard the term "leading while bleeding." It came from a T.D. Jakes pastoral conference. The title alone ministered to me. This was what I had learned, what I had been doing, and it was what I was living. Within two months of my husband leaving, I was spearheading and directing a full-blown musical at my church, directing over thirty people. I was definitely leading while bleeding. Even in writing this book, I cannot tell you how many times I just thought to myself, "What in the world makes me think that anything will ever come of this?" I had to make a commitment to write every night. Maybe the purpose of crisis in our lives is to keep us so occupied with ourselves that we do not have time for the God stuff. But now, the God stuff comes first, and the mess is secondary.

This past weekend, I heard Mario Murillo speak, and a couple of things happened as I watched him preach. First, I saw myself preaching, and then my spirit bore witness to the call. This was not the first time that something like that happened. When God first asked me to write this book, I saw myself receiving instruction from Joyce Meyer. In both instances, first with Joyce Meyer and then with Mario Murillo, I thought to myself, how ridiculous, I could never achieve such greatness in the things of God that would warrant a private audience with a woman of such caliber, and most certainly, I could never compare myself to a Mario Murillo.

However, this time God said to me, "Well, where do you think they started? Where do you think they all started?" Mario was talking about our inability to stick to commitment, and my pastor had been speaking about our inability to finish or follow through on commitments. Any way you cut it, my losses far outweighed my wins. I knew it was time to take the lead. It's not just about having a winning attitude, it's never that simple, it's about having a winning life style. Starting with your owner's manual; if you want to skip the cute name, fine, start with the Bible. Add a little, no, a lot of prayer, and then throw in some praise and worship because real Christianity is a full-time, life-long commitment. It's about always striving to make the right choices.

Do not be willing to compromise; it's never worth it. A friend of mine who has been on a diet told me this past weekend at a party that she gave up mayonnaise because the indulgence was not worth the price. We were just talking about food. Can you imagine where you would be if you took your life with Christ that seriously?

Every mistake I have made was by my own choice; I've always held the power to choose right from wrong, and when I made the wrong choice, which happened a lot, I would tell myself that I was willing to pay for it. I felt that the indulgence was worth the price. I was so very wrong because I had no real understanding of the huge price I was about to pay. If you're not going to take your own life seriously, then no one else will either. Your life just ends up being like a series of bad diets that end up failing, and in the process, you're a little worse off every time. You become a casualty of bad decisions. I definitely know that I cannot afford to waste one more day of my life paying for my self-indulgence ever again.

I believe being raised a Catholic gave me a strong foundation in Christ. I went through all the classes and sacraments that Catholics do. I went through baptism, penance, first communion, confirmation, and holy matrimony. Still now, today in my life as a Christian, I find that there are things from my Catholic upbringing that keep me grounded.

9

Born Again, and Then What?

A couple of years into my first marriage, I became born again at a Calvary Chapel service, which meant that I accepted Jesus Christ as my personal Lord and Savior. Both Paul and I had always had questions about our Catholic faith but we were busy with our own lives, so we just left it at that. We went to church if there was a funeral or a wedding, and that was pretty much it. So when I became a Christian, my complacency about Christ remained the same as when I was Catholic. I still did not go too much past that experience at Calvary Chapel.

I did not follow the experience up with church or studies about Christianity. I just kept on living life, basically trying to be a good person, yet still doing as I wanted. I kept God as an acquaintance instead of my personal Lord and Savior. I was unaware that Jesus took work; I thought everything that Jesus was offering just automatically kicked into action when I said yes to Him.

My second husband was a self-proclaimed evangelist who traveled the United States preaching and ministering to youth by the hundreds. I think that is one of the things that threw me so off about our circumstance. I would watch this guy preach his socks off, and kids would turn their lives completely around, and they would start living for Jesus, but when we got home, and the audience was gone, Michael was just simply cruel to me. By him taking advantage of my self-worth issues, I was made to feel that he meant more to God than I did, and that was why I would be treated so badly. I did not realize that it was all a show; none of it was real. So with him playing the part of the "anointed one," I left all the God stuff to him, which also made it easier for me to deal with or, actually, not deal with his backward way of Christianity.

I did not agree with most things he said, but listening to it year after year was so draining and was wearing me down. Once he was silenced in my life, it felt great just taking an untainted, deep breath of fresh air. In this debacle of a marriage, I was more like the maid that cooked and cleaned up after him and his friends. I guess you could say that I thought I could ride on his coattails of Christianity.

I made the most common mistake I think a lot of people make and that is thinking that somehow, as Christians, we are exempt from horrendous things happening to us. That is just not true; I speak from experience. I have actually found that the more productive you are in the things of God and in bringing forth God's kingdom, the more susceptible you are to disaster. You do not even think about prevention, because the thought of things happening to you just does not exist. I saw it for others but not for myself. If you do not take your relationship with God seriously and put in the work praying, reading the Bible, attending Bible studies, and attending a church regularly, it will not go any further, or should I say, deeper.

It's as if you become enrolled in the School of Christianity when you accept Christ. We all start in preschool; as you grow and learn more, you advance to kindergarten and then to first grade and so on. You have test after test, and as you pass them, you go higher and higher in grades. Many people drop out. Some are held back. Yet others do so well they get to skip a grade here and there. It is all in your hands and in your heart as to how far you want to go in life. Some will go to a junior college, while others will transfer to a state university, and yet others will go to an Ivy League school. Some will get a Master's degree and others will get their PhD.

You get the idea. Its not just about accepting Christ, it is about becoming a knowledgeable, spirit-filled, life-giving Christian.

When the Lord showed this to me, He told me that I had been stuck in junior high for years. I had failed test after test but that in the last two years, something had clicked in my spirit; I became responsible for my own Christianity and was growing by leaps and bounds. I was putting in the work and was getting great results. I was learning to live in a Christ-like way and was actually applying it. In the midst of disaster, I found I could still pass a test.

In fact, I was passing test after test. The Lord told me that I was now a senior in high school and that this book was to be my senior project. Joyce Meyer, Mario Murillo, T.D. Jakes, and Benny Hinn are just a few examples of people who went all the way with their education in Christ and received their PhD in Christianity as well as receiving their PhD in relationship with Christ. I believe that these people truly know God and vice versa. I want head knowledge as well as heart knowledge of Christ. I guarantee that when people get this far in their ministry, they must always be on their guard because that spiritual PhD also assures you a top spot on Satan's hit list.

What does that mean? It means that when you accepted Christ as your Lord and savior, it's almost as though you stepped into a supernatural boxing ring, yet I, for whatever reason, did not realize that. I was like a boxer who stepped into a ring and yet never even knew it. I wasn't even prepared to put my hands up to defend myself. The higher you go in the ranks, the harder the fights. In the beginning, everyone gets ranked as a mere amateur; the fights may not be very big, and from time to time you might even win a few. Remember, in our humanity, taking Jesus Christ out of the equation, we are conquerors. But with Christ ...

Romans 8:37: No, in all these things we are more than conquerors through him who loved us.

In our humanity, it is purely instinctual for you to defend yourself, but as we progress spiritually, the opposition seemingly gets bigger and stronger. Your true opponent is not the circumstance that stands before you; it is Satan, and he will not be as gracious as Oscar De La Hoya and fight by the rules; he will be more like Mike Tyson, who will viciously bite your ear off with his savage-like teeth. However, I have learned to rely on my cornerman, God. We need to be obedient and not only listen to our cornerman but to also put his direction into play. God gives us everything we need to win, but my arms were full of the stuff that God did not give me, which made it impossible for me to pick up what God had tried to place at my feet. I'd refused to put the stuff down, and then I blamed God, and let's not forget the devil, who works overtime to take you out.

The devil comes to kill, steal, and destroy ... everyone! In order to fight the devil, you must recognize that he is your enemy, not just to some people but to everyone. My second husband Michael considered himself to be a God-anointed evangelist as well as a blessed singer, yet even he was confused about what he perceived as attacks on his life and on his calling. He once told me that he could not understand how on the one hand, he could help so many people, and on the other hand, be so destructive and such a curse to others. The difference in being a curse or a blessing in someone's life is moving in God's will as opposed to moving in your own will.

When moving under the anointing of God, only His goodness, power, and all of His blessings will flow right through you as if someone had turned on a fire hose. However, as in the case of my second husband, when someone moves in a flesh anointing, which is often mistaken for God's anointing, it most often goes to their head. Because they are moving in the flesh, they often take credit for a move of God as their own, and worse yet, they have their own agenda but try to play it off as God's.

Remember, God will not be mocked.

Galatians 6:7-8: Do not be deceived, God cannot be mocked. A man reaps what he sows. The one who sows to please his sinful nature, from that nature will reap destruction, the one who sows to please the Spirit, from the spirit will reap eternal life.

This explains the difference between living for God and living for self. It also spells out in one simple sentence: A man reaps what he sows. That is straight, direct, and to the point, yet it is probably one of the most overlooked scriptures to this day. I know for myself, that if I had taken just this one scripture to heart, it would have kept me from harm on so many levels and instances.

In the book of Numbers, I read about a donkey:

Numbers 22:28-30: Then the Lord opened the donkey's mouth, and she said to Balaam, "What have I done to you to make you beat me

these three times?" Balaam answered the donkey, "You have made a fool of me! If I had a sword in my hand, I would kill you right now." The donkey said to Balaam, "Am I not your own donkey, which you have always ridden, to this day? Have I been in the habit of doing this to you?" "No." he said.

After God used that donkey to talk to Balaam, the donkey was still a donkey. The fact that God used her didn't change who the donkey was. Then in the book of Exodus, I read about God using a bush to speak:

Exodus 3:2: There the angel of the Lord appeared to him in flames of fire from within a bush. Moses saw that though the bush was on fire it did not burn up.

After God used that burning bush to speak to Moses, it was still a bush. God using the bush did not change the type of bush it was; the flames didn't even burn it. So too, after God uses man to minister the kingdom of God, man remains a man. We do not become better than other people; God loves us all the same. God loves my husband and his girlfriend just as much as He loves me. I had to keep reminding myself of that. It is what helped me stay clear on where I stood and kept me from thinking that I was better than them. To be respected and admired is one thing but to be worshipped and followed sounds more like a ministry of self. Being a person of great character takes work on your part, which will include embracing the characteristics of Christ. Because Christ is love, let's look at the love chapter in the Bible.

1 Corinthians 13:4-8: Love is patient, love is kind. It does not envy, it does not boast, it is not proud. It is not rude, it is not self-seeking, it is not easily angered, it keeps no record of wrongs. Love does not delight in evil but rejoices with the truth. It always protects, always trust, always hopes, always preserves. Love never fails.

What I like to do is put the name of Christ right in the scripture. Christ is patient, Christ is kind. Christ does not envy, Christ does not boast, Christ is not proud. Christ is not rude, Christ is not self-seeking, Christ is not easily angered, and Christ keeps no records of wrongs.

Christ does not delight in evil but rejoices in the truth. Christ always protects, Christ always trusts, Christ always hopes, Christ always perseveres. Christ never fails. Then I like to say it putting my name in it, and when I do, I am quickened as to what I need to work on.

Who you are as a person is on you, and so are the decisions you make. My second husband Michael always would say that he did not care what people thought and that he would not be governed by the thoughts or opinions of others or by what they might say. The problem with that way of thinking is that if we, as Christians, are to go out into the world and be a light for the entire world to see, we must also understand that we will be held accountable for being a false witness. We are to be a sample of the example, Jesus Christ. As Christians, we do not have the freedom to live however we like, not if we truly have given our lives over to Jesus Christ.

We must also always be careful not to take credit for God's work; we are no more than a vessel which God moves through. That is the mindset that I would like to adopt. I want to be pliable in God's hand but keep my feet on the ground. I lived with someone who was in the habit of letting the Anointing of God go to his head, and I witnessed the mass destruction that type of arrogance leaves behind. I have also experienced the ramifications that come with operating a ministry of "Self". Knowing what I now know, I realize staying focused as well as humble does not just happen; it comes with a price. It will cost you time and effort, blood, sweat, and tears. Overall, it will cost you your life.

What does giving your life over to Jesus Christ mean to you? We've heard that many are called but few will go all the way. How far do you want to go? What grade are you in now? I once heard Mario Murillo say that when he was going to preach his first big sermon of ten minutes, it had taken him all morning and all afternoon of the previous day to prepare. This sermon would prove to be the start of his now international ministry. If you put in the work, God will bless it. However, if you try to just get by, then that is exactly what you will achieve; you will just get by.

If you pour yourself into the things of God, He will pour Himself into you. I want to know who I am in Christ. I am tired of living a life of recovery; I want to live a life of prevention. Is it better to prevent cancer or to recover from it? Is it better never to touch drugs or to recover from drug addiction? Is it better to avoid sin or to recover from the ramifications of sin? I have now chosen to live a life of prevention.

10

Addiction Can Consume Anyone

You must learn to recognize the traps that the devil will set up for you to get caught in. I never knew that someone could become addicted to another person. I'd always believed that addictions were related to drugs and alcohol, shopping, or food. The one reason I'd never tried cocaine was because I knew that I had an addictive personality, and I was not willing to take that chance. During my first marriage, Paul was always gone, working as a police officer. At nineteen years old, I had left my home of security, and my parents as well, only to be put in an apartment that was five cities away and left there all alone. I missed my husband so much that I needed to do something to occupy my time. Two of the things I chose to help fill the void left by Paul's never ending absence were smoking and alcohol, as well as nightclubbing with friends, which I did to an excess. I even feared that I might be an alcoholic but when I got pregnant, I was able to stop both smoking and drinking from one moment to the next.

After the birth of my son, I did all right for a while in dealing with the continued absence of my husband and with the loneliness of being basically a single parent. After about six months, I started back up with smoking and an occasional night of drinking; however, unbeknownst to me, my next severe drug of choice would be Michael my second husband. If only I had taken the time to read the writing on the wall, I would have just kept right on walking past him.

Michael was abusive to me fairly early on in the relationship but I thrived on his possessiveness because the bottom line was, I felt wanted, and I was certain that I could fix the violence in him. So began my addiction. There is absolutely no good aspect of being addicted. *Webster's New World Dictionary* reads as follows:

Addiction: to give oneself up to some strong habit.

An addiction, if not broken, will eventually become life altering; whatever it is that a person gets from the addiction, it's always temporary, which in turn perpetuates a continuous need for more. What the addiction gives you is also artificial and becomes your main focal point. Everything else can fall away as long as you can get your fix of whatever it is you have surrendered your will power to. In the beginning, the list was endless as to what I was willing to walk away from to keep Michael. The addiction completely took me by surprise, and just like an addict, once I was hooked, I started to die a little with every passing day.

Once God intervened and helped me kick the habit, I finally accepted Michael's leaving, and I looked at the first year away from him as being in rehab. I stayed away from unnecessary conversation, and I most certainly did not want to see him. I actually felt myself going through withdrawals as well as real physical pain. I went to the hospital twice for what appeared to be a heart attack or anxiety attack, but I say it was a broken heart compounded by a broken spirit. I had never experienced a broken spirit before but you cannot describe it or even compare the condition to a broken heart. A broken spirit far exceeds any pain I had felt thus far.

Now that I was a recovering addict, it was of the utmost importance to stay clean. My estranged husband was leaving approximately twenty-five messages a month on my cell phone, consistently, every single month, for over a year, but I would only respond to those messages that concerned my kids, which were maybe two a month. I did everything that I could to not be pulled back into my addiction.

Michael had been gone about fourteen months, and I thought that I was doing pretty well with being over him. As long as he was out of sight, he was out of mind, which was not easy to achieve because his new life and his love interest were always around me. She worked in the same shopping center as I did, and when Michael left me, being that he worked for my father, he lost his job as well, so of course the only place he could think of getting a job at was with her, at a food establishment, which was about 150 yards from my place of business in the same strip mall.

So to avoid having to see them together or hear about them from everyone I ran into, I found a new market, new nail salon, new cleaners, basically a new complex. I would never walk out the front of my store, I always came and went from the back door. This new girlfriend also lived in the same condominium complex as I did, and once again, the only place he could come up with to move into was with her, one block over from me. So I would have to drive by their place a minimum of six times a day because they lived near the entrance of the complex.

In addition, we must not forget all of the helpful people who found it necessary to call me every other day to report the "husband with girlfriend" sightings. Most of the friends that were around during our marriage were his friends and part of "the ministry." We were supposed to be one big, happy family, all for one and one for all. However, when Michael walked away from me, they all walked away right along with him. I once heard one of them say that they did not want to take sides. Trust me when I say that I was not looking for them to take sides, but I thought just taking a stand would have been nice, you know, being a family and all. It felt as if our lives were being flushed down the toilet, and all of his friends just sat by and watched it happen, all the time being witnesses to this tragedy and saying nothing, not even so much as a call to see if the kids and I needed anything, which we very much did. When Michael left, he gave me absolutely no money for the first six months, then it was very little and sporadic after that.

These were guys whom I believed in and poured my heart into for years. I had always kept a respectful distance from the guys, because I was a married woman and because it would drive Michael insane for me to get near anyone. When ever I did sit next to someone he would give me a simple head bob which meant move now but I was always supportive from a distance. I always gave these guys a place to stay, to eat, to relax, and to socialize and, in some cases, to live. My thinking was that I was taking care of God's soldiers, and I believed in what "we" were supposed to be standing for, which was Jesus Christ. It just seemed to all get lost in the mix. This was a bit painful, to say the least.

In all fairness, there were two women who kept reaching out to me with phone calls and a letter or two. I would just listen to the messages and read the letters over and over again, but I was simply unable to reach back. I guess it was because I considered them to still be connected to my husband, and at that point I wanted all ties with him severed. It sure did make a difference, though, at least to know that someone cared enough to reach out and that they saw me as a person. For years I had watched all the guys in "his ministry" go through different relationships. I watched the girlfriends come and go and even a wife or two, but I never thought that the kids and I would ever end up on that list of exes. I ended up on the never-to-be-seen-or-heard-from-again list. However, God reminded me that the seed I planted into these lives was on God's behalf and that I was to look to Him and not man for my return. My blessing would come from God. Not man.

The kids and I changed our whole routine so as to not run into any uncomfortable situations, and I was starting to feel as if I was able to deal with things and feel O.K., maybe even let my guard down a little. Boy was I slapped back into reality when my husband decided to send his girlfriend to my house to bring us groceries. You have to understand that I had not spoken one word to this woman, who knew my children and me for some time before she even met Michael.

She knew us well enough to know that when she saw us drive up to the restaurant, which meals to fix and how we liked everything, so it was a bit disturbing knowing she knew that he was my husband when she went for him. I slowly pulled around the corner to my house as I watched her unload the car, leaving bags of food at the door and then drive away. I was at a complete loss for words and infuriated; I had been reduced to accepting groceries from the woman my husband left me for? The worst part was that I had to take them, because I needed them. I walked up to the house and made my kids get the groceries into the house as quickly as possible because my second emotion after being infuriated was embarrassment.

I immediately called Michael and asked him if there was no limit to his stupidity. He had the audacity to deny even sending her to my house; my daughter and I were sitting in my car watching her, and at the very same moment, he was on the phone saying that he had left the groceries himself. I felt a gripping of my heart and then God spoke to my spirit and said, "Did you forget what I showed you?" I instantly remembered the night I found his car at her house. "Who told you to let your guard down? No, there is no limit to his stupidity. Now hang up the phone and dust yourself off. We are not losing any ground today." So I did; I put the groceries away by myself and through prayer, I actually found that I was able to be thankful for the food. To be very honest, Michael's girlfriend had done a pretty good job. While I was putting the groceries away, I realized that she had also done the shopping as well. I could tell by the brands and type of food that was bought. My husband couldn't even do that task on his own.

It is funny how sometimes we pray to God for help and then complain about how He gets it to us. This little ordeal did mess with me for a while but then I thought, hey, the girlfriend is the one who got the short end of this stick because my husband sent her to go to the market and buy his wife and children groceries. Instead of feeling like, "That's what she deserved," I felt horrid. My husband had moved in on her life and conquered and consumed her as he did with me years earlier. Michael moved in on her place of business, moved into her home, and was even driving her brand-new car. Remember to watch out for those takers.

11

Just How Long Is This Addiction Going to Last?

A week after the grocery incident, I saw Michael at a school function. I watched him walking through the crowd, talking to this person and talking to that person; he was shaking hands, kissing cheeks, and giving hugs. Part of me wanted everybody to hate him for what he had done to me but that went against everything I was now standing for and embracing.

"Standing" sounds so easy, but at times it can feel like you're standing in a twister like Dorothy in *The Wizard of Oz*. These people hadn't seen him for over eight months, and it seemed like he was right at home and I was once again the outsider. That's not how it was but because of my insecurities, his presence made me feel that way. Kind of like that puppy that gets beaten repeatedly and tends to cower instinctively when the abuser steps towards them. I also felt the same way I had felt for all those years of being with him when I was always on the outside looking in, always wanting to be a part of his world but I was only allowed to watch from afar. I felt sick to my stomach just being near him. Not that his presence made me sick because of what he had done to me, but because I felt myself starting to cower.

I kept trying to smile and look unaffected but I could not figure out what was wrong or what was making me feel sick. I kept my distance but he just kept coming towards me. I had managed to stay clear of him up until the end of the program, when I was backstage getting my girls. He came up from behind and caught me off-guard. He completely invaded what I would call my personal space. He would step in, I would step back, he stepped in again, I stepped back, and then he leaned in, placing his hand in the middle of my back to prevent me from moving again, and he whispered right into my ear, cheek to cheek, "What are you doing? Don't pull away from me."

Then it hit me like a ton of bricks. I was still addicted to him. I still longed for him. I still missed him. I was stunned. Oh my Lord Jesus, how in the world is that possible? I felt my face get red and flushed, and I felt the river of tears starting to break through. I moved away as quickly as I could, because there was no way I was going to give him the satisfaction of knowing that he could still affect me that way.

The questions that were flooding my head silenced everything around me so that all I could hear were my questions to God. Why in the world won't you take this from me? It makes no sense, it is not fair, it is just not fair, I did what you said, when you said, "WALK AWAY," I walked and I let him go. I have not looked back, not even once.

As I stood there in complete shock and disbelief, I became so very depressed. So sad, so disappointed, so alone. Needless to say, I learned that kicking an addiction is much more than walking away. You must take back your power. If you don't take back what you gave up in the first place, which is your will power, you leave yourself open to be ambushed by your addiction when you least expect it. Remember…

Addiction: to give oneself up to some strong habit.

I wasted no time in getting back into a rehab state of mind. I worked on repairing my heart, my spirit, and my will. This incident at the school function just made things clear as to where I was. I had to understand that when I felt like cowering or when I felt that he still had a hold on me, it did not mean that I was failing; I was just not as far along in my recovery as I thought. Those feelings just confirmed that I still had some work to do on this particular project. It took me quite some time before I could even admit to someone that I was still addicted to him, because I was so embarrassed. The question of me still loving him had been posed to me on many occasions. To be honest, I was unclear of the answer. I would cleverly sidestep the question but leave them thinking that I absolutely did not. I wanted the answer to be no, but I was not sure; I had not yet learned the difference between love and addiction.

I then started to work on the new vision that God had started in me. One of the many things that God had told me was that I was to go out into the world as a women's advocate and teach women how to overcome this mental and spiritual rape, but how or where do I even start? How was I going to teach women something that I was still suffering the effects of? I could not comprehend when people would say things like, you are so beautiful, you are so talented, you are so gifted, or you are a phenomenal mother; it just didn't match with the image that I still saw in the mirror, which was an aging, unattractive woman. I now have an understanding of a symptom people who suffer from anorexia experience and how what they see in the mirror and believe in their hearts is the furthest thing from the truth, and yet the truth does not change what they see.

I remember one day going to church and many people had very overwhelming compliments, like, "You look so gorgeous," for example. Half of those compliments were from people I had never even spoken to but had seen every Sunday for years. That day I was approached by at least twenty people who felt compelled to come up to me and express themselves. I felt flushed and just wanted to hurry up and get to my seat. You see, that which was supposed to make me feel phenomenal made me feel uncomfortable, as if I were a spectacle, because the praise did not coincide with what I saw in my own reflection. Therefore, I saw all of their compliments as a bad attempt to try and make me feel better about my horrible situation.

When I was sitting in church, waiting for praise and worship to start, a good-looking man sat down next to me. I became very uncomfortable. I looked at how unattractive my hands were, so I hid them under my Bible. Then, I saw my feet and thought, "Oh, my God," and I remembered how many times Michael had made mention of my unattractive feet, so I hid them by tucking them under my seat. I had not realized just how damaged I was. I still believed everything negative that I had been fed by Michael for all those years.

Whether it was physical, mental, spiritual, or financial, I had lost everything as if I went up in flames. I was burned down to the ground. When someone has their house burned down, it does not matter if it was an accident or not, it does not matter that they are sorry, it does not matter that everyone who stood by and watched it burn is crying with them: THE HOUSE IS STILL BURNED DOWN. I was living in a burned-down house.

The problem was that I had not fully assessed the damage. What does assessing the full damage mean? The first thing to do is get a hold of your insurance provider, and trust me when I say this, there is no better insurance provider than God. Unlike Farmers, All State, or any other worldly insurance provider, all God requires from you is for you to reach out to Him, and He will send the best of everything. It will not be automatic. You must take the first step and ask for help before God will move. God told me, on many occasions, that everything I had lost was completely covered. Not only was everything covered, but also that He was going to give me over and above anything I had thought or hoped for, starting with my self-respect. I noticed that once God was able to get my complete and undivided attention and Michael and I were apart, my metamorphosis began.

I saw the movie *Peter Pan* with Robin Williams. There was a part in the movie when one of the lost boys came face to face with Peter Pan but did not recognize him because life and Peter's choices had physically changed him and altered who he was. The little boy reached up, putting his hands on Peter's face, and moved his face around. He moved it side to side, up and down, and then he moved it back, and much to his surprise, he'd seen enough traces of who Peter used to be to recognize him. Then the little boy said, "There you are, Peter." As I sat in the movie theatre, tears came to my eyes, because I realized that I, at that moment, also recognized that person I'd let go of a long time ago.

I was experiencing a freedom that I had voluntarily surrendered to a man over and over again throughout my life. I was no longer trying just to fit in or to not be annoying to someone. I was actually able to experience the things that I liked and enjoyed without constantly being put down for my choices. However, I did have to battle my mood swings, which were major. The bad ones would always come when I was alone. I would tell myself that I was going to use the time for prayer but I would always end up in tears, in the dark, soaking my pillows again with tears that I had already cried. When I would experience these down times, it only helped the distorted pictures of the way I saw myself come and distract me yet once more. My eyes would swell, and my complexion would get blotchy, and I would even start overeating again. Then I would start with the other woman junk, and how could I ever compare to her nonsense, and so the cycle continued.

12

It Was Time to Expand My World

It took me until 2004 to get the Internet and an e-mail address but I finally got on-line service in my home. I was telling my brother how fascinating I found this Internet world, and he told me that if I really wanted to feel insignificant, I should do a Web search under my name. So one night when I could not sleep, I got up about 3:00 a.m. and ran my name. There were many, many extraordinary women with my name; I was just not one of them. This in turn started the whole I'm-so-worthless thing up again.

Out of curiosity, I decided to run a few names that I found to be intimidating. First I searched Ed Traut Ministries. There were 113 different items on him. Then I searched Frieda White Ministries, which had 277 different items. Then I searched Mario Murillo Ministries, with 876; Joyce Meyer Ministries, with 2,190 items; and last but not least, T.D. Jakes Ministries, with a whopping 10,200 items. So, what was I supposed to get from this?

Establishing yourself is a progression, a process, a way of life. Part of walking in the fullness of your anointing and your calling is to allow God to transform your mind, heart, and soul. Only then can you reach the depths of what God has for you.

Although these people experience greatness through God, there is no telling how much even they are unable to tap into because we all fall short, everyone! There is not even one perfect human being; we all have faults, and seeing ourselves for who we are in our humanity is essential. If we were going to judge anyone, we should start with ourselves, because if we are truly honest with ourselves, this should stop us from throwing stones. To be honest, I have had many stones in my hands these past two years. Most of them I picked up in retaliation of Michael's actions, and all of them were picked up with hatred, venom, hurt, and anger. I was fighting not to let his actions pull me into his arena, which is exactly what the devil wanted. It took a lot to drop them one by one, especially since I felt that the world was just waiting to see the destruction I would cause once I heaved them. I found as I started to drop them that my burden lightened because I found victory in not going the way the world said to go but going the way God said to go. I went to the Bible for help.

Romans 12:17-19: Do not repay anyone evil for evil. Be careful to do what is right in the eyes of everybody. If it is possible, as far as it depends on you, live at peace with everyone. Do not take revenge, my friends, but leave room for God's wrath, for it is written, "It is mine to avenge; I will repay," says the Lord.

Once I had learned to drop the stones, I had to learn to not even pick them up. Besides, being preoccupied with all those stones was just another way for the devil to keep me busy on his plans rather than God's plans.

So with that bridge crossed, I started working on myself and on seeing God's plans for my life. God kept giving me glimpses of things that He wanted to get done through my hands. We are talking astronomically big things. However, God told me to keep these revelations to myself because now that the ball was in His court, he could finally work through me. He said, "Just be pliable in my hands."

Jeremiah 18:5-6: Then the word of the Lord came to me, "O house of Israel, can I not do with you as this potter does?" declares the LORD. "Like clay in the hands of the potter, so are you in My hand, O house of Israel!"

The things that God would bring to my attention were awesome, yet disturbing, but I did not care, I wanted to see all that God had to show me. He gave me dream after dream and vision after vision. The following is just one of the things that God wanted to get started through me. It is a letter that I felt compelled to write to Oprah Winfrey.

Dear Oprah,   October 25, 2004

Three or four weeks ago, I saw your show about the abusive husband that allowed his behavior to be taped by your cameras. As I watched the couple sitting on your stage, I was in a state of shock. My spirit bore witness to this woman's pain. It is so incredible how through you and your resources, we are able to witness the worst as well as the best in people. You open yourself to God and you have become a strong weapon in His hand. That is what I strive to be. The can of worms you opened on that show has been sealed far too long. I pray that your spirit bears witness to what I am about to reveal to you because ever since that show, God would not leave it alone. When that woman came back on your show for a follow-up, there had been no change in her. She is now just the shell of who she used to be. He should be secondary at this stage of the game.

She suffers from a disorder that I need you to help me bring to light. I recognized myself sitting there next to you on that stage. For the past year and a half, I have been working on recovery from this disorder that had no name. After the show, I kept praying for the Lord to show me what the whole purpose of 13 years of abuse was for. I kept asking, "Lord, what is it? What is it called? I can see it but I can't make out the name." So, I started trying to find out the name, all the while knowing that I was not going to find it.

I have been seeing a counselor for the past 3 months. Her name is Stephanie Wagoner. She is a certified marriage and family therapist. She also has her Master's degree in human services. I was mainly trying to get help for my kids but ended up getting much more than I had bargained for. A week ago, I arrived for a session with Stephanie. Before I walked into the office I looked back at my parked car, recently damaged in a car accident. A bungee cord held the hood closed, electrician's tape held the lights together, the front quarter panels and grill grimaced back at me in a distorted mechanical sneer. I wondered when I would have time to take it in to be fixed. As we began our session Stephanie sought to help me to accept the damage to my life as she had done in her own life years earlier after also having come through a destructive marriage. It was then that God told me that like myself and my car, Stephanie had only stopped the process and had not taken the time to go back to "fix" the damage. God told me, "Tell Stephanie that this is what she has done to herself. She is praying that I will help her accept and embrace the damage but I want to FIX it. I want to overhaul everything so that she is better than ever before." Only Stephanie can tell you what she thought about my revelation, though I am sure that it gave her some clarity. When I went to pay for the session I think she thought that she should pay me.

So, with that, I left to let God deposit the rest in her Himself and went back to trying to get the name for the disorder. I had told some friends that I was trying to figure out something big that God was trying to get to me. I had a sense of urgency because not hundreds, not even thousands, but millions of lives are being affected daily by this disorder. You know that a high number of women die at the hands of their husbands? Over half of them, had they had a name for it, may have been able to get the help they needed. Then one morning, it flowed out, like a fire hose that had been turned on. Here it is. In its raw state.

Adam's Rib Disorder (ARD)

This is a disorder specifically inflicted on women, by their husbands. The cause can include but not be limited to mental, verbal, emotional, spiritual, and physical abuse, likened to repeatedly being raped. This disorder, if incorrectly diagnosed, will lead to the woman being diagnosed as anorexic, clinically depressed, having low self-image, or being suicidal. This in turn can lead to unnecessary medicating, which only compounds the problem and her well-being. What makes this condition so hard to identify is the woman's overwhelming need to protect her husband. Secrecy is essential for continued diminished capacity. Her greatest problem is her love for him. His greatest strength is the same, her love for him. By the time her love dissipates, she is too weak a person to get out by herself. Every fiber of the person she represented has been ripped away little by little until she can no longer recognize who she sees in the mirror. If undetected, she can ultimately be mentally, emotionally, spiritually, and in some cases physically murdered. If children are involved, they too experience the effects of this man's abuse. Once ARD is established, the husband must be removed from the situation immediately. In the same way that he would be removed for child abuse, he needs to be removed and stopped from inflicting any further damage on his wife. She has proven herself incapable of protecting herself or her children and needs intervention. The first concern should be the stability of the woman's environment. Saving the marriage is secondary. The fact that the husband has been able to do this only clarifies that the marriage was over quite some time ago.

I realize that this sounds like it goes against most Christian beliefs but on the contrary; it is about saving her life. Once her life is stabilized, the rest will come together like a ripple effect. Sustaining emotional, mental, or physical abuse from your husband was never part of the deal. This is taking "for better or worse" off the charts, overboard.

The problem you will run into is that her views are completely distorted. The same way an anorexic sees a fat person in the mirror, the ARD patient's view is all out of focus. The next step is getting her to understand that she is blind to reality. Her understanding that her view is distorted does not change her view, but gets her into the correct fighting stance. Stopping the abuse is only half of the solution. The damage must be reversed. If not, she will live the effects of this disorder for the rest of her life and most likely run into it again because she will never feel worthy of anything better. The effects on the children are the same. They have been taught the same distortion. Their love for the abusive father now becomes a downfall to them because either they do not want to see wrong in him, or they completely go the other way and never want to see him again. Both cases are detrimental to the child. Therefore, we must work at correcting their distorted views as well, in turn stopping the vicious circle. Instead of becoming Adam's Rib, you become "A dam rib."

Deborah A. Cosio
Author

Oprah,

I am a survivor of this disorder who is looking to be a conqueror of it. I am actively working through my distorted views of who I am. I keep telling myself, "What I see in the mirror is wrong." And pray that one day it sticks. For now, I walk in the power of knowing that it is wrong. Despite all the voices that tell me the hundred and one reasons why I should not waste my time with this, I move forward with it. When you shine the light on this, you are even going to hear from mothers who lost their daughters to this. They are going to say, "I knew that it was something, I just couldn't put my finger on it. But I now know that my daughter died as a result of ARD." It is the most empowering thing to know you are not worthless or crazy. I am not a scholar or a doctor. I do not have a PhD. What I do have is a PhD in surviving this disorder and a willing heart, and God told me that that is all He needs. With God's help, I will make what I have gone through worth it. Help me get this recognized as a real and living disorder. I keep thinking about that woman that was on your show. I cannot get her out of my mind. She is the one who needs the help. He needs to get the hell out of there so that first, the damage is stopped and then the healing can begin. She said it from her own mouth that she was afraid. The tears would not stop and she could barely raise her head.

I saw the show when you gave the cars away. I saw the show when you threw the world's largest baby shower. I now can see the show that has half an audience of women who fit in this category and half an audience of female therapist ready to get this revelation and then turn to help these women to "see" when you turn the lights on. God bless you and your people for all the work you do on bettering lives.

This particular experience took five days to completely manifest itself, and I must say that it was actually exhilarating. Although the outcome is not what's most important, my willingness to obey is.

13

Communication with God
Is Essential for Success

Having an open line of communication with God helped to make my situation easier to understand. I had been battling, and with good reason. I had allowed myself to be put through hell. Why I allowed it is irrelevant; it was still hell. However, the key word is "through"; I'd made it out. Yes, I was very ragged and torn up but out just the same. Then God revealed to me why my second marriage was never going to work, and He asked me to pick up the Bible.

Genesis 2:18-22: The Lord God said, "It is not good for the man to be alone; I will make a helper suitable for him." ... Then the Lord God made a woman from the rib he had taken out of the man, and He brought her to the man.

God then gently spoke to my spirit and whispered, "I said it is not good for man to be alone and then I brought him woman. I brought man woman, singular, not many women. I did not say to rifle through this bunch of women. I did not say that when you get tired or it gets too hard, to move on to the next woman in line. I brought him woman. I brought him flesh of his flesh and bone of his bone. Every time Michael abused you, he was in fact causing self-mutilation." When God put it that way, everything made sense. It was as if the devil thought to himself, "Hmmmm! If God himself said that it is not good for man to be without woman, then to kill, steal, and destroy man's soul and his God-given destiny, I will have man destroy the one thing God said he needs: woman. In this way I will take out two birds with one stone. I will kill woman through man, in turn killing man, and as a bonus, I will get to his seed as well."

As this revelation began to seep in to my spirit, I thought to myself, "I think not." As far as I am concerned, this bird is still very much in flight, and as for my seed, they are all three doing well and growing stronger than ever in their lives. I also came to understand that it was not Michael's heart or drive to become what he had become in my life or what he had become in the lives of my children. He had never learned and was unable to learn, up to this point, what it was to be a good man, to take care of and nurture your wife and your children, to be a Godly head of household. Could he learn in the future? Absolutely. We all have the same God-given potential.

However, it will cost him because he will have to do just as much, if not more, soul-searching work as I have had to do, and still, I am only partially there. Not only did I have to recover from fifteen years of various abuses, I also had to heal from the horrific way Michael decided to end our relationship, his continuous disregard for the kids, me, and our living environment. Then, as if coming out of a coma, it hit me. All the things that I was suffering at the hands and actions of Michael were the very same things I had done to cause my first husband, to suffer by my own hands. I was no better than my soon-to-be ex-husband number two. Somehow, I had managed to block that part out of my mind. I had somehow talked myself into believing that I'd had a good enough reason to leave my first husband and you know something, maybe I did, but not the way I did it. I'd made myself believe that I had every right to walk out, to change my mind, to quit, but now I see that I was so very wrong.

You hear it every day: "You reap what you sow," "What goes around comes around," "Treat others as you would have them treat you." The Bible only gives you two ways out: infidelity and abandonment. I had been unfaithful in my first marriage, and now I was being handed the same bitter pill, yet I could not bring myself to swallow it. The Bible does not say anything about if you're not getting what you need from your spouse, or if you get tired of him, or if you feel unloved, to go out and find someone else who does make you feel loved.

I had spent the last year and a half pointing the finger at Michael and his girlfriend, when I had done the exact same thing to someone else thirteen years prior. In fact, I was worse than my second husband and his girlfriend because I thought that somehow I was better than them. I actually saw myself as better than my second husband, when in reality, he was just my reflection in a mirror. A mirror that I would be forced to look at so that I could then look back and see, feel, and answer to what I had never been held accountable for. It was time to face the music; it was time to face what I had done and who I had become in the process.

Now that I had this reflection in the mirror to deal with, I knew I had to face it head on in order to change it.

I began to evaluate the past year and a half, and I finally understood exactly what I had done to my first husband. It was hard to not loathe myself for causing such pain to people in my life but I was not to loathe myself; I was to learn and grow, so that my reflection in the mirror would be changed. All I know is that I had to keep moving forward no matter how bad I felt about who I had become. Whether I was walking forward, falling forward, or crawling forward, it was always in the same direction. Slowly but surely, my reflection began to change. My kids and I were excelling at a rapid rate, not just in the healing process but in all areas of our lives. For the first time ever, both my girls had made the school honor roll. My teenage son, from my first marriage, was in a church play, had landed the lead role in a high school theatre production, and played starting defense on his junior varsity football team all the while managing to carry a B average on his report card. I was writing a book, directing plays, on the school board, offered a position teaching acting, running my parents' business, monitoring my father's health, and taking him to all his appointments.

We were attending church two to three services a week, tithing consistently, because all of us were striving to finally put God first. The girls had counseling, tutoring, piano lessons, voice lessons, guitar, dance, shows, field trips, auditions, rehearsals, and doctors and dental appointments. All of this was on top of your basic mom jobs like cooking, cleaning, washing, homework, playing referee between the kids, being a sounding board and a hero. I was somehow making this happen while I was at the lowest point in my life; I had just been completely devastated. I cannot even begin to imagine what I could be capable of at the top of my game. I realized that I had to stand back and reword what I was thinking. It wasn't me; it was God. I'd finally allowed God to become my strength. I was living "When I am weak, He is strong." God was the reason for the flying colors in our lives. He is the only explanation for our growth, healing, and grace.

The day after this revelation was a Sunday. I went to church with a smile from ear to ear. I felt confident, strong, empowered, and enlightened. The reflection in the mirror had changed for all of us. My next lesson would be not to get too caught up in the hype of feeling great but to first learn balance. Too much of anything can be bad and will eventually cause a shift to the extreme, thus causing you to be out of balance. I had never realized just how off-track my life had truly been because balance was something I had never strived for. I did not know how essential it was until I started experiencing the fullness of joyous moments and then I would nose-dive instantaneously.

Well, on this particular Sunday, somehow, a man whose name I did not even know was able to verbally come against me in a way I was not prepared for. Looking back on it now, he seemed to be trying to defend himself in regard to something that he might have been contemplating or felt guilty about himself. He insinuated that I had driven my husband into the arms of another woman, and that just sent me running from the church in tears, before church was even over, and had me sitting in my car crying. I cried on and off about his insinuation for two days. I cannot remember ever being talked to like that, with the exception of my husband Michael, of course.

I sat in my car and asked, "God, how could a man that I do not even know cause me to react like this? How can I go out into the world for you, whether it be to preach, teach, or just plain minister to people, when a nameless, faceless man can hurt me so badly?" And God said that it was time to work on developing a thicker skin. He began the transformation at my home church so that I could work on it around my family and friends. Instead of letting things reach me personally, I must learn to minister to people. This man at my church did not know me personally; therefore, it was not personal. God told me, "It is no longer about you; it is time to get over yourself, so that I can use you to help others. Now! That is enough! It is time!"

I found that I had unintentionally ended up milking my "poor me," victim role. In addition, my family and friends unintentionally made it easy for me to stay there. It made me feel good and cared for to have everyone hugging me and giving me the "poor you" treatment. I was starving for any kind of attention as well as affection. I was playing the needy card; thus, I once again ended up relying on people instead of God. This was hard stuff to get through my head. Just when I thought I had it, I didn't. The whole point is that I wanted to live for God. I had lived for my husband, my kids, my dad, my mom, you name it, and I lived for it. One of the hardest things for me to swallow is that "man," no matter who he is, has the potential to leave you. We, as humans, are as imperfect as they come. Yet, that is whom we tend to put most of our trust in. What if we put our lives in God's hands? What if we put our trust in God? He is the only true guarantee.

Deuteronomy 31:8: "The Lord himself goes before you and will be with you, He will never leave you nor forsake you; Do not be afraid; do not be discouraged."

God's word states that He will never leave you nor forsake you. Although we would like to believe the same about the people in our lives, there is just no guarantee. Living for God is very demanding and calls for a disciplined life. However, I do know that anything worth having is worth working for. I was determined not to be beaten again by putting my trust in man. For years, I had blamed Satan for all of my downfalls. I blamed him for all of those "attacks" when, in reality, Satan was rarely involved; he rarely had to be. Actually, he did very little. My free will choices were what took me down most of the time. I was doing Satan's job for him.

14

Be Actively Assertive in Your Life

God gives us free will. This gift or privilege of choice can be one of our greatest assets or one of our biggest downfalls. I was still straddling the line; I was not doing bad things but I was also not making successful choices that would help me to move on. I was merely treading water. I do not know if you have ever treaded water before, but eventually you do get tired. If you were out at sea, treading water, waiting to be rescued, and no one came, in time you would inevitably drown. So instead of just treading water, I became actively assertive in pursuing my life, or at least what I wanted to make of my life, which was and is to make a difference for the better, wherever I am. Free will is only an asset when it is properly applied in our lives. Furthermore, it can only be applied by one's self. What we say and do, what we eat, what we read, what we choose to listen to, what we watch, and how we react are all aspects of our free will. It is all a part of who we are and where we are going in life. God will guide us but we have to do the work; we are responsible for making the right choices.

For instance, God gives us the armor we need to fight any and all battles, but we must choose to put it on ourselves.

Ephesians 6:13-17: Therefore put on the full armor of God, so that when the day of evil comes, you may be able to stand your ground, and after you have done everything, to stand. Stand firm then, with

belt of truth buckled around your waist, with the breastplate of righteousness in place, and your feet fitted with the readiness that comes with the gospel of peace. In addition to all this, take up the shield of faith, with which you can extinguish all the flaming arrows of the evil one.

The first three words are "Therefore put on…" Not "Let me dress you" or "Let me help you pick it up." God will not dress us; we must do it ourselves. We must read our Bible, pray, praise Him, worship Him, and we must fellowship with God on our own. Just going to church is absolutely not enough, not if we desire a deeper relationship with God. Our actions mean everything; I know it sounds cliché, but actions speak louder than words. If you speak it, follow through with what you say, and then you will actively see it come to pass. If you say, yes Lord, follow through when you hear His voice, plain and simple. Even if God asks you to write a book, then be obedient and write it. If He asks you to direct a play, then direct it; if He asks you to offer money, teach a class, take a class, or minister to people, then just do it.

One of the greatest gifts that the Lord has given me is the ability to hear His voice. For years, I longed to just hear a whisper. I used to say to myself, oh, if I could just know God in that way, on that level, I would be so joyous. Once I was able to focus and hear His voice, I fell in love with Him on a completely new level. For years, I'd envied Michael because I believed that he had a special ability to hear God's voice. I remember one time not too long ago, when my elder daughter was having some fear issues. She wanted to stay with me instead of going to her dad's house because when she would feel gripped with fear, we would just stop and pray, and she didn't know if her dad knew how to do that. When she told him why she wanted to stay home with me, his response was, "Don't you know who I am, don't you know that I have a direct line to God?" I explained to her later that we all have that direct line to God. I realized that it was years and years of comments such as those that kept me thinking that somehow a person needed to have a special "anointing" to hear God's voice, which I thought my husband had, and that it was not available for the rest of us "un-anointed" people. I would pray night after night, "Lord, why won't you speak to me? Please, I want to hear your voice so desperately." So, when it did not happen, I became satisfied with being blessed enough just to be around and care for God's favorite ones such as Michael and the guys under him in "his ministry." I thought that Michael was more important to God because he said that he could hear God's voice and I could not. I saw myself as less in the world and less in comparison to my husband, so why wouldn't I be less to God? I had allowed one man to get me so twisted in my way of thinking.

Know this as fact: God wants you to hear His voice. He would absolutely love nothing more than to have an open conversation with you, but you first must learn how to listen. You must be open to hear Him through whatever venue God chooses. Whether it is the mountains or the ocean, the wind or the rain, in torn-up roots in your back yard or in your own child's words, just be open to His voice. You'll see that things become so much clearer and completely awesome in just knowing that you are worthy in God's eyes. Assertively pursue the voice of God. As I said before, it is one of my most cherished, God-given gifts. And don't fall for that woman's intuition stuff, that is God. The world feels more comfortable putting that label on it but don't fall for that another day. It is the voice of God, through the Holy Spirit, speaking directly to you. Have you ever said, I don't know how I knew, it was just a feeling. That feeling was also the Holy Spirit.

Although I had been massively damaged by Michael and had come to the realization that he had not even been a friend in my life, I chose to forgive him. If I wanted a true chance at surviving this divorce, I had to release all the emotional poison. I had never sustained this much destruction from anyone in my life, much less someone I had been desperately in love with. Yet I still offered the same grace to him that had been bestowed upon me by God, as well as by family and friends years earlier in my life when I had committed the same offenses. I had been married, had an affair, left my husband Paul, broke up my son's home and family, and later married the "other man, Michael." Your first instinct might be to say, "Well, I would never ...." If that is what came to your mind then you have just set yourself up. Maybe not now or tomorrow but when you least expect it, expect it. If you are of the human species, then you are capable of mistakes. When you can admit that you are capable of making mistakes, then you can work on preventing the mistakes. Remember, it is better to prevent cancer than to recover from it.

Becoming aware of your gifts is essential for maximum effectiveness. Then you must understand the fullness of your gifts and abilities. Let's take free will; in its raw state, it is like a wild stallion that has not been broken, running wild and aimlessly, fighting any and all opposition, without reason, with no understanding of rules, even causing itself harm in the fight of rebellion. The stallion must be broken. If not, he will never be useful. You will continuously be thrown and land in all kinds of messes.

This got me thinking about all these things that I was supposed to be doing in my life and why it was that I couldn't seem to get more than a thing or two going at a time. I saw this special on cable about a man named Andrew Van Buren. He is recognized as the number one plate spinner in the United Kingdom. He has standing sticks and spins china plates on the top of the sticks. I saw as many as twenty-one plates spun at one time. When one would start to fall, he caught it and started it up again, and if, by chance, one hit the floor and broke, he simply reached for another. He did not stop to cry over the broken plate but quickly set his sights on the new plate. Once he got them all going, he had only seconds to stand back and admire his accomplishment, and then it was right back to catching and spinning again. It took complete concentration and precision.

Now, look at everything we need to take care of in life; see them all as plates that need to be spun. I am good at spinning three or four plates at a time, but the problem is that I have about twenty-one plates that need to be spun at one time. When I get three or four spinning well, I sit back and have a coffee break, admiring my work, but because of my position, when the plate falls, I am too far away to catch it, and it hits the floor and breaks. Nine times out of ten, I sit and cry over the broken plate as I pick it up piece by piece. I concentrate on my failure rather than just picking up another plate and spinning it. It's really not any more complicated than that, yet we make it harder than it has to be. Go back to basics, back to your ABCs. Get your broom and dustpan, sweep it up, and throw it away; just get rid of it and start again. Sometimes, we can be our own worst enemy. There is nothing worse than being a "know it all" in trouble. Can it be that simple? Absolutely, it can, and is. If you can dream it, and see it, you can make it happen.

Then, I started recognizing everything that I was touching was someone's completion of thought, dream, and determination. In order for it to get to my hands, someone had to see it through. The laptop I am using at this very moment started out as an idea in someone's head; they saw it through, and the laptop came to be. The paper I take notes on, the pen I use to make those notes, the chair I am sitting in, even the ankle socks on my feet. It can be a dizzying thought, but just stop for one minute and look around; literally, do it. Every single thing you lay your eyes on is the completion of someone's thoughts, dreams, and vision. Everything!

I think about how many ideas and dreams I have had over the years that never came to pass; we are talking about a full graveyard of ideas and dreams that I let die. Yes, it may have been accidental but the results were still the same: death! I let plate after plate drop, just smashing to the ground. Don't just go through life stumbling through it like I did. Only you know what is inside of you, and no one can live out your dreams but you. So live life intentionally. Name your plates and start spinning. From cooking dinner to doing laundry, working, raising kids, dieting, exercising, writing a book, even directing a play; from spiritual multitasking to just knowing who your God is.

I have many plates to spin in my life. I will no longer just sit and watch them, wish for them, or think of them, but I will, with complete concentration and precision, do my best to get them up and keep them all spinning, and if one falls and breaks, I will simply reach for another. Is it that easy? Yes, it is.

Please do not misunderstand me. All these ways of looking at life are just tools to help get you to where you are supposed to go. Remember, a true Olympian must have all the right tools for proper training. They need the right equipment, clothing, diet, sleep, exercise, and coach. Having the right tools will make his training go smoother but it will still take gut-wrenching work to become part of the elite.

15

Never Compete for Your Own Children's Affections

I remember my second Christmas without Michael. I'd found out several days prior to Christmas that my husband was planning to introduce his girlfriend to our girls. I felt as if there was nothing I could do about it because Michael usually did whatever he wanted regardless of how others felt. So, I would have to deal with the idea that on Christmas, they would all be together for the first time. I was quite aware that our marriage was over but I could not help feeling that it was the worst thing in the world to do to my girls. It was as if he was planning on dunking my girls in a tub of cold water, with ice cubes. Why on Christmas? Why take the chance of scarring them for life on such a big holiday?

Apparently, the two of them had gifts for the girls. Five days before Christmas, my estranged husband eased them into the whole situation and let the girls know what was going on and that they would meet his girlfriend on Christmas. Of course this was without any warning, but the girls seemed to be fine; yes, they had a few tears, but overall, they appeared to handle the news well. I, on the other hand, was showing signs of major stress. From the moment he spoke to me and let me know what he was planning, I was battling my flesh. I wanted to cause him pain, give him a piece of my mind, cuss him out, or slash his tires. I even thought that if he died in an accident, it wouldn't have been the end of the world. I remember every time I saw a special report on the news, I would watch with great anticipation that possibly it would be him. That is the God's honest truth. I am not proud of those thoughts but they did exist. Within the first two days, I had bitten off all of my fingernails to the point of not being able to touch things without pain, and I was back to crying in my pillow at night.

I went and spent money that I most certainly did not have on Christmas presents for my girls, over $500; I know now that it was in an attempt to outdo whatever Michael and his girlfriend were going to give them. It was as if, on Christmas, after a year and a half, I was going to hand over my entire family to the other woman. "She" would finally succeed at getting them all, but the hardest thing of all is that they would all be together and happy and I would be all alone.

I was eating like a maniac and losing all sight of any beauty I had struggled to reclaim. The ugly woman in the mirror was back, and she was uglier than ever. I always say that actions speak louder than words, and I was searching for the right actions to fight this battle within myself. The first thing I had to do was recognize what was going on. It took me a few days because I'd thought that all I was worried about were my girls, and this really was the main focus of my concern, but I also came to realize that I was not ready to swallow yet another pill being forced down my throat, which was the other woman. Why couldn't he seem to do any of this divorce stuff in the right way or order? Then my past came to mind; I didn't wait or do things in the right order when I left my first husband for my now-second husband, Michael; what goes around, comes around.

All this time, I had blocked out the girlfriend's name. I don't know if I had intentionally forgotten it; remember, she was friends with the girls and me before she became involved with my husband, but when my husband came to see me to go over the details, thereby assuring himself that I wouldn't foil his plans for a Merry Christmas, he just blurted out her name for the first time ever. I remember how just the sound of her name made my body cringe, and my head popped back as if I were being sucker punched right in the face. *Webster's Dictionary* defines it as an unexpected punch. I thought, "Beautiful; could this woman get any more real to me?"

You would think that I would have learned to be more careful with my questions, because when you ask God, God is faithful to answer. It took about fifteen minutes after removing the ton of bricks my husband had just verbally dumped on me before I could even move. As soon as I gathered myself back together, I began praying for my husband and his girlfriend. At first, I did not know what to pray for although, now, I at least had a name. Then it hit me: I would pray, YOUR WILL IN THEIR LIVES! Hey, if it worked for me, then it must work for everyone. I went to church and prayed for them.

Don't get me wrong, it wasn't as though I was asking, "Lord, may their life together be blessed." I still hadn't gotten that far yet; it was simply, "Your will in their lives." I felt that I could not go wrong with that. There is no way to taint that prayer, and if there were, you would really have to go out of your way to find it. At church, I had given an offering in the form of monetary seed because, no matter how I felt, I was determined to not let the circumstances manifest negatively in my life, and for this reason I gave on their behalf. I remember asking myself, "Why write about it?" Everything I had learned in church said that these things should be done in secret.

Matthew 6:1-4: Jesus said, "Be careful not to do your acts of righteousness before men, to be seen by them. If you do, you will have no reward from your Father in heaven. "So when you give to the needy, do not announce it with trumpets, as the hypocrites do in the synagogues and on the streets, to be honored by men. I tell you the truth, they have received their reward in full. But when you give to the needy, do not let your left hand know what your right hand is doing, so that your giving may be in secret. Then your Father, who sees what is done in secret, will reward you.

So back to my original question of, why write about it? The answer is simple: Because I am to become a women's advocate and I am to teach. These are not mere words on a page. You have heard the phrase "Do as I say, not as I do"; well, my phrase is "Do as I do." Because I have lived through it, and I stand as a living testimony that it can be done God's way. I was in the middle of directing an original play for my church, which was to be presented as a New Year's Eve dinner theatre production, and I was not about to let this interrupt my work for the kingdom.

While in the midst of taking a stand for the kingdom of God, something amazing and life altering was transpiring within me. I decided that I was no longer going to try to buy my own kids. I was not going to compete with anyone for my own flesh and blood. If I could not afford to lavish them with gifts, so be it. If they were blessed by other venues, then so be it. I would move in the opposite direction of where my flesh was pulling me. If I was up crying at night, I would get out of bed and would write or clean house instead of wallowing in depression. Whatever ploys the enemy raised up to tear me down, I began to use them to build myself up and, in turn, further the kingdom.

My request to Michael was that before my girls meet the other woman, that he wait until the divorce was final. His response was that we were as good as divorced. He assured me that all the papers were in and it was now just a waiting game. He found my request for him to wait for the divorce to be unreasonable, and he was not willing to hold off for the final papers. At that point, I decided to put myself in spiritual, mental, and emotional restraints. I had to finally take a stand and make decisions as head of my household, and based upon what I felt was best for my children as well as myself, I decided not to allow my girls to meet his girlfriend on Christmas Day. I was not going to take the chance of it being a disaster on a major holiday and engraved in their memories forever as well as put myself through that particularly unpleasant event. Some might have called it selfish, which maybe it partially was, but I like to call it mental survival and cautious damage control.

16

When God Says, "It's Time," It's Time!

By the way, the New Year's Eve dinner theatre was a big success. The dinner part had a few glitches, but the play itself received outstanding reviews. So much so, that two weeks later, the church would bring the play back for another performance.

It is possible to fight our battles even in the midst of our storms: God's way. It will, however, take great concentration and focus. Many people react first and then think later. The problem with that is we are human, which makes us fallible. Believe me when I say that most of the decisions I have made in the past two years went against my natural or human grain. I am not a super human. I wanted to do and say many things that went against my Christianity, yet I chose not to because I simply grew weary of doing things my way and always coming up with the short end of the stick. I was determined not to go for the quick fix and embarrass myself by reacting to what I was being faced with. The whole point of the Bible is to use it as a guide for living.

We are to use it all the time, not just when it suits what we feel. The Bible does not give us free license to react any way we want. We, as Christians, are to follow Godly principles. So let's just start with the basics: the Ten Commandments:

<u>*The Ten Commandments given to Moses are these:*</u>

<u>*1. You shall have no other gods before me.*</u>

<u>*2. You shall not make a graven image.*</u>

<u>*3. You shall not take the name of the Lord your God in vain.*</u>

<u>*4. Observe the Sabbath day by keeping it holy.*</u>

<u>*5. You shall not dishonor your parents.*</u>

<u>*6. You shall not murder.*</u>

<u>*7. You shall not commit adultery*</u>

<u>*8. You shall not steal.*</u>

<u>*9. You shall not give false testimony against your neighbor.*</u>

<u>*10. You shall not covet your neighbor's wife.*</u>

Yes, I know we are not perfect but I also know how easy it is to use that as an excuse. We might say to ourselves, "Hey, I am only human." Somehow, we feel that that gives us the right to go off and do some pretty outrageous things.

Even though I did not permit Michael to introduce the other woman to my children on Christmas Day, eventually the day did come. It was the day after New Year's. The girls were to meet their father at the mall; however, he had conveniently failed to mention that his girlfriend would be joining them. I knew in my gut that something was up when he asked me to drop them off at the mall entrance and that he would be waiting for them just inside the door. I knew in my heart that this was the day.

I saw no reason to fight it any longer because sooner or later, Michael would do what he wanted, divorce or no divorce. I just prayed, "Lord, be with me, help me, console me, do not let me act out in the flesh, do not let me make things worse for my girls." I knew they were going to be fine because before the girlfriend had gotten involved with Michael, my girls liked her; we all did. That was what I should really have wanted; if my heart and concern was truly for my girls, then what else could I ask for? I truly believe that "actions speak louder than words," so if my main concern was for my girls, then wouldn't it be better for them to feel great about her as opposed to not liking her and being miserable every time they were with her?

So why did it crush me when I heard my girls singing her praises, when I heard them tell me how cute and nice she was, and when they said it went great? I will tell you why: Because if my husband of twelve years liked her better than me, then they too could like her better than me. That is what my insecure, poor self-image was screaming back at me in the mirror. It took every ounce of self-control for me not to make them feel weird or bad because they truly enjoyed being with her. I sat there with the most convincing smile and gave them the impression that I was just great.

The older one said, "Mom, look at me in the eyes so I can tell if you're all right." I just stared straight ahead, gripping the steering wheel so tightly that my fingernails dug into the flesh of my palms and my knuckles turned ghostly white. She repeated, "MOM, I need to know that you're all right. I'll know if you're all right if I look in your eyes." So, with the biggest look of love I could muster, I pulled over, turned, and gave her a great big smile. I even threw in a chuckle for good measure and then, with a deep sigh of relief, she was good. Inside, it just felt like another slap in my face but this time at the hands of my own children. I do not know why I took it that way. I did have quite a few choice words for him that wanted to leap out of my mouth but I just kept swallowing them, one after another. I refused to call and verbally vomit all over him.

When we got home I wanted to go upstairs and lock myself in my room. However, I purposely sat with my girls and watched cartoons in an effort to play it all off. The T.V. was blaring, the kids were laughing, and my son was on his computer writing, yet all I heard was a deafening silence. I felt as if I were deaf or watching a silent movie or, better yet, stuck in a nightmare, moving in slow motion, and could not wake up. I searched my mind for someone to call and unload on but could not think of anyone. Besides, if I were to do that, then I would lose this battle. I felt that if I were to strike out in any way, I would be giving this situation power over me, so I just sat there in silence and prayed for strength. I knew that Michael was probably pacing the floor anxiously while waiting for his phone to blow up with my call, and he did not know what to make of it when it simply did not happen.

I'm guessing that he could not take the suspense any longer because a couple of hours later, he managed to come up with a lame excuse and showed up at my door without notice, which was something he'd agreed never to do. He was dropping off some of his girlfriend's used clothes for one of my girls, which included a pair of pants and a sweater, to be exact. I thought, "GOD, please do not let me react; I have come this far without losing it. So what if he brings my daughter the used clothes of his girlfriend?"

I just took them and said thanks. He then asked me to step outside for a moment. I guess he could not wait any longer to be blasted by my mouth but I just could not do it. He seemed to be at a loss for words, as was I. I know he spoke kindly but I cannot tell you what he said. Either it did not register or maybe I was still in that deaf mode. Although he was trying to strike up dialogue between us, I did not want to engage in any conversation. I simply assured him that the girls were fine. I made it a point not to give him my take on the situation. He hadn't taken my feelings into consideration earlier in the day, so why act concerned now? And truth be told, I really didn't want to say anything that would either bring him down or set him off. This was one of the things that needed to be stopped. When we were living together, we seemed to feed off of each other in that way. Making each other feel pointless or brainless seemed to be what we had become best at; it had become our main ministry.

I also realized that about five years ago, when Michael and I had agreed to try to work together and get our marriage back on track, I had made the decision to forgive him for the abuse of the past. Please understand that I willingly made that choice, or so I thought. The problem was that I did not realize that my forgiveness was conditional. We did not restart on an even keel or as equals. You can say you forgive someone but how many of us truly forget?

When God forgives us, it is as if it never happened, never to be brought up again. Can you imagine how life would be if whenever you made a mistake, God brought out your track record? So, that is how we lived for a couple of years. I was the forgiving wife and he was the husband trying to make it up to me. He would be the one indebted to me for staying and I would be the one reminding him of all the things that I had to endure because of him. He was the one trying to catch up, and I was the one keeping score.

That is not a marriage, it is a prison sentence. He became the defendant and I became the prosecutor. We should have been one, working on our future together, not him paying for his past mistakes and me always reminding him of how unfulfilled I was.

It was a horrid existence on both parts. There were no winners. He was never good enough, and I was never happy. All the while, we were missing the "now" part of life. The next question I had to ask myself was, "Would I ever get it right?" I wanted so badly for my life to mean something, not to be a waste. I can tell you, though, as long as you have breath in your body, it is never too late to get it right. Furthermore, not everything in my life was a waste. While even in the midst of all my screw-ups, God was still able to use me in some ways, just not to the fullest.

Do not misunderstand what I am saying; I'm not trying to downplay the severity of my actions. Two failed marriages is a big deal, I know. However, I've asked God to forgive me and I stand forgiven, as if it never happened, the way we are supposed to forgive. I take full responsibility for my own damaging decisions. I am truly sorry that I failed in making the right choices. I am sorry for the sadness I brought into the lives of my first husband's family, my second husband's family, my kids, my family, and an endless list of friends. I know that I cannot take it back or undo it.

Once I started to realize how many people had actually been negatively affected due to my horrible decisions, I was stunned. One might say, "Oh, she is just being too hard on herself." Well, I am guessing that had I taken the time to thoroughly think out the ramifications of my actions, things might have ended up much differently.

17

If You Have to Hide It,
Chances Are, It's Wrong

Here is a good way to tell if you are about to make the wrong turn: If you have to keep it a secret from your family and friends, chances are, it is wrong. This me, me, me world I ended up in, is a very selfish and self-damaging place to live. I can only promise the people in my life today, that from here on out, I will think before I act, speak, react, or respond. I will live to fulfill God's purpose in my life, not my own. I trust that God will take care of me. I have learned that the best defensive strategy for me in the midst of battle is not to put all my effort into fixing my own situation. I will leave that for God. Instead, I will put my energy into God's work, which will in turn give me the ammunition I need to stay strong while God does His stuff in my life. Do not worry about not having a place in God's plan; God always has work for you. He will line up your duties but first you must say, "Yes Lord."

If the situation looks impossible, good, that means God's getting ready to shine His greatness through you! I cannot begin to explain that feeling that I get when I finish or complete a work for God. To use the word "Awesome!" is an understatement. It is one of those things you will have to experience for yourself. With every page that I write or production that I direct, I feel a great sense of accomplishment and great strength in knowing that I am a mighty weapon in the hand of God, even in the midst of my storm. It does not matter what I sometimes see in the mirror because what I tend to see is a lie from the pit of hell.

I reject those negative images, and I choose to remember that my view can be somewhat distorted. God says that I am the head and not the tail, I am above not beneath, and I am more than a conqueror. The list of how God sees us goes on and on. I choose to believe that God's list of who I am is the truth and put my list, which is the lie, under my foot along with the devil's head. I will not allow the devil to have power over me or my calling.

You must purpose the desires of your heart. My will is strong, I will go as far as to say, stronger than the average person's. When I was twenty-four years old, I feared that I had become an alcoholic. (Remember when I talked about filling the void of my first husband's absence with other things? The nightlife was one of those things.) I was going out to nightclubs at least four to five times a week. Drinking happened to be a big part of that scene; I also smoked about two packs of cigarettes a day. My concern grew stronger when I decided to get pregnant. My heart's desire became having a child, so I stopped everything cold turkey the day I was confirmed pregnant. After my son was born, I returned to moderate drinking and smoking just one pack a day. It was normal to me. It was a way of life. I had grown up at a time when smoking and drinking was socially acceptable.

I myself started smoking in the eighth grade. Both my parents smoked, and it was definitely part of the nightlife, which I was still occasionally engaging in. Then when my twenty-seventh birthday was approaching, I decided that I had had enough. I set a goal to quit smoking on my birthday. I was not going to let a cigarette have more power over me than my own will. So, thirty days before I turned twenty-seven years old, I was getting ready to kick the habit. I embedded the idea of quitting in my mind and embraced it as a heartfelt desire. I was back up to two packs a day and was getting in all the smoking I could before the day. When that day hit, I never smoked again. Not even one puff. Eleven years into smoking and I just walked away from it from one day to the next. Now if that is not strong will, I do not know what is.

All humans have the capacity of a strong will. The strength of your will is not what is in question. It is the strength of your desire that gets most of us in hot water. God says, "I will give you the desires of your heart." However, the desires of my heart are what led me into getting so off-track and wrapped up in sin.

God keeps his promises; the desires of my heart were self-centered as well as self-destructive. Just because someone wants something that does not mean that they should get it. We have rules and regulations that we should abide by. Do you remember the Ten Commandments? Think about every time you got off-track; was it possibly because you broke one? Reckless living hurts you as well as all of those involved and those who love you. Hurting people is a high price to pay and pretty irresponsible, to say the least. I am guilty of living this way in the past but my future will be quite a different story because I now understand the concept of the desires of the heart.

We must purpose and protect the desires of our hearts. When we find ourselves in situations that compromise or go against what we know is right or go against what we are embracing as a heartfelt desire, we should just get up and get away from it.

One wrong turn is all it takes to get lost. The devil's sole purpose is to kill, steal, and destroy, to get us to turn left when our God given destiny is on the next right. It is as if one day I got on the freeway going south when I was supposed to go north and never noticed. It does not take long for us to lose sight of our dreams, and unless we get off and turn around, we will never get to where we are supposed to go. I had gotten so far off-track that when I finally did turn around and was headed in the right direction, I did not even recognize my dreams as renewed. I thought that they were all brand new, as if they had never existed before. A writer and a director, are you kidding? A public speaker, Come on now!

Then one day while I was cleaning, I opened a drawer and accidentally came across some old videos that my first husband Paul and I had worked on twenty years ago. At first, it was just fun to watch them with my kids; they were very excited. They said things like, "Oh my God, you were so full of life," and "You were so cool." It was as if I had been suffering from amnesia and then the lights suddenly had come on. I was watching myself, twenty years ago, acting, casting, directing, and producing. I remembered that I'd started writing just out of high school when I went to college and took a writing class, where I would write in my journal daily. I was also affiliated with an acting group through Paramount Studios and spoke many times in front of large groups. How could I have forgotten all of it? It was my passion, my drive, my gift, and I completely walked away from all of it. I got on the wrong freeway, and I just kept on going blindly, aimlessly, in the wrong direction. It was all my choice. I allowed the desires of my heart to be altered, I let my guard down, and the devil had a field day with my life and the lives of all who were connected to me.

So now what? There is definitely a choice to be made if you come to this crossroad in your life. Do I get hung up on the fact that I just lost twenty years of my God-given destiny or excited that I found my way back to it? I say that I have no more room for negativity in my life and choose to look forward to my future.

18

My New Year Would Bring a New Nightmare!

It was a New Year, and I was expecting great and awesome things in this "New Year." I had survived the girls meeting the girlfriend. I had twelve days until my next performance at the church, and I knew that many new people would come to see the play. Rehearsals were going well and everything, for this one day, was calm. Then it started up again. What I thought was over had actually just begun. The year and a half that I had just survived was only a preview of things yet to come. The feeling of peace that fell upon me was to be short-lived; unbeknownst to me, I was merely in the eye of the storm, and the roughest weather was still ahead.

I found out that Michael never filed his side of the paperwork, so my divorce was not as close as I'd thought. Finances once again came to a standstill, and I had just added a $412 medical insurance bill to my plate. Hey, that's not too bad, with my past year and a half, not a problem, or so I thought.

It was a quiet, cool Saturday morning and I was lying in my bed, with the window open and a gentle breeze caressing my skin. I was listening to the birds outside as I was praying and thanking God for being so awesome in my life. Thanking Him for showing me how to deal with catastrophe with dignity. I was proud of myself. Then God, literally, physically pulled on my sleeve, to the point of causing me to turn and see who was next to me on my bed. For a moment I thought that one of my girls had come into my room, but when I saw that there was no one there, I slowly laid back down on my bed and crossed my hands on my stomach.

Then God spoke to me, He said, "Oh, by the way, we have one more thing we need to take care of. It will take immediate action on your part. You cannot go around this. You must go through it. I will lead but you must follow. Step where I step and keep your eyes on me. Do not look to your left or to your right. Just trust in me and who I can be in your life." Then, without any thought, with my left hand, I slowly reached over and put my hand on my right breast, and immediately I felt the problem. I immediately removed my hand with a gasp of air, and I knew instantaneously what I was touching.

In the past, I'd had lumps in my breast, in fact in a fifteen-year period, I had three lumps removed without any problems. I had been doing yearly mammograms for eight years but when Michael left, I had let a lot of things get away from me because I was so distraught and it just so happened that my yearly mammogram was one of them. So I was very familiar with the feel of my breast, and this was definitely not like anything I had ever felt before. As a matter of fact, I couldn't even remember the last time I had felt my breast for any type of lump. For a moment, I curled up in a ball in my bed and thought, no, no, no! no! NO! NO! Please. That is enough! What happened to my "New Year"? What happened to my new life? I do not understand. How in the world do I go through this one alone? I am still alone. Have you forgotten that I still lie here, night after night, in this bed, all alone? There is no one here to help me, to hold me, to take care of me. I have no covering. I have no husband. And once again God said, "I am here. I will help you. I will hold you. I will take care of you. You do not lie here night after night all alone. I have always been here. Always! You are MY bride."

In Hebrews 13:5 God said, "I will NEVER leave you nor forsake you."

In *Webster's Dictionary*, I looked up the word "never." **1. Not ever; at no time; 2. Not at all; by no chance; in no case; under no conditions.**

God said, "I will never leave you." He used the word "never." God's word is an all-or-nothing deal. You are not given the option to pick and choose from the Bible what you are going to believe today and then tomorrow decide that it does not work for you. I find it amazing that nine times out of ten, when hit with a crisis, that is exactly what we end up doing. Is it hard to live by the Bible? At first, absolutely, without a doubt, but as time passes, it becomes a way of life. It will always take focus and concentration but is better than the alternative, which is our own way, I do not know about you but with my past record of accomplishments, I am done playing God. I stink at it.

Remember, it was my tendency to first find someone, usually a man, to latch onto in a time of crisis, and it had not fully become natural to me to latch onto God first. Once again, my first instinct was to reach for man but this time I did not react without thinking it through. After a moment, I laid back on my bed, took in what God had just said, took a deep breath, and latched onto God. I said, "All right, let's go." I sat up, took a deep breath, and just went about my day. I walked without fear or anger. Maybe I had nervous knots and definite sadness, but this time, this crisis, things felt different. Change will always feel different, and you must give it a chance to set in. I did not let Satan riddle my mind with fear, doubt, or a spirit of death. I went to church the next day and praised and worshipped God just because I love Him, not to get something in return.

First thing Monday morning, I wasted no time and started walking through. I let my dad know what was going on so he would know where I was going to be and so that he could cover me in prayer. I was in the doctor's office by 9:15 a.m. as a walk-in. I wanted to say, "I cannot believe that I am here, alone, doing this." Then I heard God say, "I am right here."

The doctor came in to give me a breast exam and while he was feeling my breast, he said, out loud, without thinking, "Oh my God." His tone had shock and great concern. In my head I was thinking, "Hello, I can hear what you are saying. A little bedside manner wouldn't be out of line right about now. " By 10:00 a.m., I was walking to the mammography department, and just as the thoughts of being alone began to form in my head, God said again, "Hey, I am right here." I was put in the front of the line in mammography. The tech doing the test, which by the way was an excruciating test to say the least, just blurted out without thought or reason, "Oh my God! Don't put your clothes on and wait here."

As I sat there with tears just streaming down my face, yet once more God said, "Hey, I am right here with you."

By 11:00 a.m., I was walking the long cold hall to yet another department. I heard God say, "Hey, I am right here." I was put in front of the line in the ultrasound department. Thirty minutes later, I was signing consent forms for surgery. I was going to have a biopsy. Tears were streaming and I thought, "Oh my God, What's happening? I didn't even have time to call anyone, not even my mom." Then God whispered very softly in my ear, "Hey, I am right here with you." It was as if I could feel the warmth of his breath on my ear and neck, which caused me to turn my head. I felt chills through my entire body. Just then, the nurse reached out and held my hand very tightly. I was holding the hand of a total stranger, and I felt comfort. God was covering me through any and all means, even through the hand of a stranger.

The surgery was done with a local anesthetic and was very painful. I could actually feel them cutting small pieces of my flesh from my body. By 12:15 in the afternoon, I was driving home wrapped in Ace bandages and ice packs, saying to myself, "I don't understand, what just happened to me?" I was having trouble driving through the tears. I kept pulling over to calm down. I felt as if I had just been violated in some way. I could not reach my mom by phone. I kept thinking about my kids. I kept thinking of all those times I had thought about not wanting to go on because of a second disastrous marriage. I cannot tell you how many times, in the past year and a half, I kept asking myself if life was worth going on. How astronomically stupid did I feel now? I could not find the words if I tried. Everything in the past had become instantly insignificant. Of course, I want to live. Lord, please forgive me for being so adolescent, so self-centered, and so narrow-minded.

Everyone that I had shared my situation with kept saying that everything was going to be all right. That it was nothing. They would say that in the name of Jesus, I was healed. Now, I knew that all that was true, it was just not as simple as that. I knew that this particular cup was mine but I felt I could not share that with anyone because I did not want to appear to have no faith in what God could do, but I knew in my spirit that this would be proof of God in my life for others to see, learn, and believe. This would give me the platform to show others how to walk without fear but with faith.

The doctor told me that I would have to wait until Friday to get my results. I decided that the results that I would concentrate on would be for the number of salvations that I would witness after the play on Friday instead of whether or not I had cancer. I did not miss a step. The next day, I had rehearsal and everything went well. As I started to let people in on my secret, they were taking it very badly. I guess most people equate cancer with death. I did not know how to handle people breaking down on me. People felt so incredibly bad for me. And if they were close and knew of my life in the recent past, it was ten times worse. I found myself trying to uplift them, which really took everything out of me. I would run into someone and they were happy, then by the time they walked away, they were distraught and very sad. I went out of my way to give generously to my cast and crew because I wanted them to know how much I appreciated them and how important they were by giving me an avenue in which to battle.

That Friday night, we had twenty-nine people accept Jesus Christ, and I was elated that I could still be effective for God in the midst of my storm. That night when I went to bed, I was thinking of where I would take the play next. The thought then came, "What audacity you have. You are about to face something much bigger than you, and you are thinking about another play. Are you crazy? It is time to put you and your family first. Get your priorities straight. Get your divorce done, get your life in order, for once in your life just focus on you!"

I knew that that is exactly what Satan wanted me to do. He was trying to pull me back into that me, me, self-absorbed world that God had just helped me pull myself out of. It suddenly came to me that when I take care of God's house, He takes care of my house. Satan will mix a little truth in with his lies to make it more believable. The truth part of Satan's message was that this was going to be bigger than me, but when God is for us, who can be against us? I was not going to make the mistake of taking this out of God's hands. I decided to stay focused on my ministry while taking care of my daily responsibilities.

19

It Was Time for My Results

The following Monday, I had my next doctor's appointment to get my results. My mom and two friends Jim and Lucy insisted on going with me. I really did not think it was necessary but it seemed important to them so I did not argue. Besides, I was trusting in God and figured He was writing it out this way for a reason. I looked at my mom, and I knew she was not prepared for a negative result. She would not even consider the possibility. As she and I waited in the examination room, with me on the table in a gown and her sitting on the stool, I asked her, "Mom, have you even considered that maybe this isn't going to turn out good?" It was obvious that it had not even entered her mind; she sat back in her chair, stunned at my question, with her eyes wide open, and gave me no response.

The silence was broken by a soft tapping on the door. The door opened and the doctor came in and wasted no time. He said, "Hello, my name is Dr. Verham, and you tested positive for breast cancer." There are those moments in life that you never forget, like the first time you fall in love, the first time you make love, the first time you feel hard labor pain, the first time you experience the death of a loved one, the first time you hear, "I'm leaving you." Or the first time you set your eyes on your first child. Some experiences are quite electrifying, while others are horrifying, but there is nothing that quite describes the feeling that you get when you hear, "You have breast cancer."

I looked at my mother as all color left her face. She seemed to stop breathing for a moment and did not know where to look. I sat there completely still. Tears gently, and ever so slowly, streamed down my face. It was so quiet that you could hear the tears as they hit my gown. I was not surprised, just deeply saddened.

Instantly, I was faced with the decision of a lumpectomy or a mastectomy. What? Wait! And it needed to be done within two weeks. Mastectomy, over and done with, or lumpectomy, we may not get it all, in that case, we will need more surgery, and you will also need daily radiation for six weeks. Oh yeah, you get chemotherapy, either way. Five minutes later, all four of us were sitting in a room with a woman, hearing all the pros and cons of both options. We were all in a state of shock but trying our best to listen. I had passed the point of anything sinking in after the first ten minutes. My RAM was overloaded. I knew that I had to call some people who were waiting for the results, so while she kept talking, I was writing down a list of names and numbers for my friend Lucy to call. I also wrote a short monologue for Lucy to read to them because I knew if I opened my mouth, I would lose it. It said something to this effect:

Hello,

I am calling for Debbie; the results were positive for cancer. She is fine but she just cannot speak at the moment. She will call you as soon as she is able.

I did all that while the lady was speaking to me. Maybe she thought I was taking notes on what she was saying. Forty minutes later, the woman was still talking. Then, without warning, she plopped down and opened a book, which caused me to look without thinking, and she showed me a picture of a woman who was missing one breast. I just shot up out of my seat, slammed the book shut, and barked, "That's it people!" That was all I could take for the moment, and thank God, she finally stopped speaking. I asked her to schedule the lumpectomy. I'd decided that I was going to give God the opportunity to let me keep my breast but, if they did not get all the cancer, then I would agree to the mastectomy.

At this point, life was more important than my vanity. I somehow was moving with an inner strength that I had never known, and then I hit a wall. My intention was to put everything on hold just until the smoke cleared. However, in reality what happened was that I completely shut down mentally, and that seemed to be exactly what Satan wanted.

Unfortunately, the smoke didn't clear until three days had come and gone. When I finally came out of my comatose state, I called my church to speak to the administrator; I let him know the situation and that I was not going to let this stop me in my ministry. I admitted that it might slow me down for a moment but it would never, ever stop me. He was careful with his words but he let me know that another church had called about the play. They were interested in an encore performance, and he wanted to know my thoughts on the subject. Considering what I had just been hit with, it would take some work to keep it together because two of the main cast members had suddenly left the ensemble, yet all I could say was, "Yes, let's do it!"

I did not have to scramble for a minute. I just kept walking in God's footsteps. I did not look to the left or to the right. I personally explained to my cast and crew that there would be times when I'd come to rehearsals directly from chemotherapy and that I might be exceptionally rough around the edges, but they all seemed to know that God was giving me the room that I needed to battle, and they were all in for the long haul. As far as the cancer was concerned, I read up on just what I needed to and dealt with things as I got there. The lumpectomy was the first of those things, which, by the way, also included the removal of eight lymph nodes from under my arm to test if the cancer had possibly spread.

The doctor explained that if I wanted to, I had the option to go home the same day of the surgery, and I said, "Absolutely, yes, I will want to go home." You know how tough we like to think we are? Well honey, let me tell you. When I started to come out of the anesthesia in recovery, I had flashbacks of major labor pains like you would not believe. I was in so much pain that I could not even fathom the idea of leaving the hospital, not to mention that you do not get to take that little morphine button home with you.

So needless to say, I stayed overnight. Everyone came in to see me to make sure that I was all right and then left me for the night. The pain under my arm was intense but I still had my breast, a bit mangled but still there. It took a while to recover from the anesthesia with all the little unpleasantries but I was a real trooper.

Unfortunately, the surgery happened to take place on my mother's birthday, and I was determined to make it up to her, so when they came to pick me up the next day from the hospital, we went straight to a restaurant for dinner. We were also supposed to go to the movies but dinner was as far as super woman could go. I had a very uncomfortable drainage tube, two different incisions, and tape pulling and tugging all over the place.

The doctor told me that it would take three working days to get the results of the biopsies, which would have made it on a Wednesday. Of course, when I called, there were no results in yet. The same went for Thursday, Friday, the weekend, and again nothing on Monday. However, Tuesday, now Tuesday would be the day. It was funny how everyone kept coming up with his or her ideas of why it was taking so long. I heard, "No news is good news." "It's taking so long because they can't find anything." I even heard, "This is just a test to see how long it would take you to curse God." I can guarantee that the last one never even came close. I knew that whatever the answer, God was with me. Yes, I was facing a giant, like David facing Goliath, but I know how that story ends.

So, with that in mind, this time I heard Dr. Verham say, "We did not get it all; it was much bigger than we originally thought. I took out a large piece but we did not have clear margins." The bottom line was more surgery. This time it would be a mastectomy. Wow! Talk about deafening silence. I sat and could hear nothing, absolutely nothing.

I was remembering about a year back, when I was trying to find something attractive about myself to start to build my confidence on. You know, there were only two things that I still had absolute confidence in as a woman: a great bust line and beautiful, healthy hair. I know it may sound shallow but that is the reality of what we face as women. Wanting to look attractive, especially now that I had no love interest, was becoming more and more unlikely to me, but then I remembered I had decided life over vanity. I scheduled the mastectomy for the next week.

20

I Received Beautiful Roses that Would Never Die

I spent most of my time trying to get my living space in order. Laundry, cleaning, dusting, but it all seemed out of hand. I was having trouble focusing. Everywhere I looked, no matter how much I'd done, I saw that there was always something else that needed to be fixed. Everything seemed like a man's job but I had no man to help me. After a couple of days, I started to panic and I called my older brother; I was so upset that I could not even speak. I just cried and mumbled a few words, and that was it. The next day, a work crew consisting of my immediate family came to my house and ripped through it in a day. They would not let me lift a finger. It was God using my family to say, "Let me do it, let ME take care of you."

I was bombarded with feelings of joy then embarrassment, thankfulness then inadequacies. When it was all over, the good won out the bad and God received all the glory. I had to learn not only to recognize God but to receive from Him as well. But in order for that to happen, I had to put my pride aside first.

It was three days before my surgery, and my elder daughter was singing with her school at the Los Angeles Children's Hospital, for kids who were long-term patients. I went to hear them perform to keep my mind off the obvious. As I walked into the hospital, I remember thinking how devastating it would be to have one of my kids as a patient in this place. What I was facing suddenly became easier; if I had to face cancer, better in me than in one of my children. As I stood in the back of the room and listened to my daughter sing these incredible notes and heard the children clapping for her, I started to get chills. God told me, "Here is a rose for you today. She is not only talented but ministers to others at eleven years of age. She is not all about herself; she is learning to care for those around her. I want you to carry this rose with you today and always know that this rose will never die."

I had been given roses before in my life but not one had ever thrilled me so as much as this God-given rose. Later that evening, my seventeen-year-old son, who was in advance drama at his high school, had his first opening night as a principal role, which was in *Noises Off.* As I watched my son perform, God would give me yet another rose in the form of my son. He said, "Look, watch him, he is incredibly talented, and he ministers to others through those talents. He has learned to bless those around him, and his fragrance is so sweet, enjoy him!"

God did not stop there; later that night when everything had calmed down, my little one came into my room with a smile like a Cheshire Cat. In her hand was a paper from school with an A++ on it. It was her spelling test, when just two years ago, she could not even read. Once more God said, "Look at how far she has come and look how pleased she is with herself. She no longer feels stupid but proud to bring this home to you. She is not tainted by your mistakes but flourishes through your example." My bouquet was beautiful and awesome to take in.

It was only two days before my surgery and yet I was beaming from ear to ear with joy; however, God still did not stop with the roses. The next morning, I received a call from my sister-in-law. She had become one of my main confidants since the cancer hit. Somehow she had the ability to stand back and see through all the emotion and help me sort things out. She asked if she could meet me at my house for a moment. I was so busy trying to take care of all the last-minute business before I went into the hospital, I said O.K., but just for a minute. Back then I was having a hard time putting food in the refrigerator because of my lack of finances, so what does God do through her? She drove up in her Yukon, full of groceries and the essentials from toothpaste to toilet paper and again God said, "Here is another rose for today. Know how important you are to me and to those around you."

What abundance! She brought big packages of food, the good stuff and the best. I was resting in the arms of my Father and it felt heavenly. There was not a person on the planet that could have given to me as perfectly and as sweetly as God did. I was in the best place that I had ever been in my entire life. The world might have said, "What could she be talking about? I wouldn't wish her past even on my worst enemy."

In *Webster's Dictionary*, I looked up the word "past." It says **1. gone by; ended; over [his past troubles]; 2. Of a former time; bygone; 3. Immediately preceding; just gone by.**

That meant that my life had just begun, and who better to be with than with God? I smiled from ear to ear all day. Anyone on the outside looking in would have thought that I was in a cloud-nine type of love, and they would have been right. That night before I went to bed, I made a point to take a good look at myself in the mirror. I wanted a clear mental picture of what someday would be again after reconstruction.

It's the morning of the surgery and I'm sure it comes as no surprise that the roses just kept on coming. My check-in time was 8:00 a.m., and I was not at all in a hurry to get there. I arrived at 7:55 a.m., only to find an army of people waiting to walk me up to surgery. It was like a bouquet of roses in the form of family and friends. I was speechless and surprisingly very joyous. But there was one woman in particular whose presence there surprised me the most. Her name is Janice Carr. Just to get to the hospital, she had to take a taxi for over an hour, and she had been waiting for two hours for my arrival. This woman had also been through some life-threatening storms, one of which happened to be breast cancer.

She is an evangelist and singer who travels the world singing and ministering. I had not really spoken to her much on a personal level, just occasionally, but I had been blessed by her vocal gifting countless times before. I did not know how to express my gratitude for her presence but I let go and let God lavish me with whatever He wanted.

As I lay in my gown and hospital bed waiting to be medicated, the nurse announced in the waiting room that anyone who wanted to see me before I went under had better go in then. They came in two by two, taking turns, two by two by two. I had more people there than I had when any one of my children were born. One might expect me to be scared and nervous prior to surgery; however, I had a great inexplicable peace. Love overcame the situation through my immediate family and my family in Christ. I closed my eyes and went to sleep.

I had told everyone in advance that it was all right to come in and see me when I woke up from the anesthesia to make sure that I was fine, but then I wanted everyone to leave and give me at least twenty-four hours to get a grip and adjust to the reality of losing my breast. That is exactly what happened. They hugged me, kissed me, and left. That is, all except for Janice, the woman who took the taxi. She sat at the foot of my bed and never left. She sat quietly, in the dark. I would occasionally wake up to vomit, ask for pain medication, or turn over, and I would see her silhouette in the shadows, watching over me. I never had to say anything; in fact, just seeing her there, kept me at peace. God's rose for this day was an angel standing guard over me, protecting me, making sure that nothing would come near me during my time of vulnerability.

During my previous surgery, immediately following the lumpectomy, while I was drugged and not in the right state of mind to defend myself, I had been visited by a social worker. She was asking probing question about my life and my children as well. I spoke of certain abuses that my children had experienced at the hands of their father (which, by the way, had already been reported to the Department of Children's Services as well as reported to the police). She insinuated that I was lying to cover up for Michael and contacted Children's Services on her own. When she realized that I was telling the truth, she came to apologize and said that she had entered my room by mistake; there was another woman in the next room who wanted to file a complaint. I told her that it wasn't a problem, but the more I thought about it, the more violated I felt, mainly because I was so doped up on morphine and I was in no condition to be questioned in such an aggressive manner. I do remember that I was in tears, telling her not to open another case. I was in no condition to open another case or to have Michael yelling at me and saying, how could you do this to me again, but she was determined to file charges. Later I filed a complaint.

This time God said, "Oh no, this time I will put someone to stand guard over her myself. I will put an angel at the foot of her bed." I am still left speechless over that.

21

I Just Wanted to Hide, but God Had Other Plans

When I came home, I was not nearly in as much pain as I was after the lumpectomy. To put it bluntly, this time they just cut out all muscle, tissue, and any extra flesh, leaving only skin. This time it was more of a mental wound than a physical one. Do not get me wrong; there is substantial physical healing that needs to take place when you undergo the removal of a breast, but it cannot even compare to the mental one.

To my surprise, people from my church had arranged to bring us dinner for a total of eight days: dinner, dessert, and drinks, the works. Instantly, I was thrown back into a position of receiving, not to mention I was forced to face people right off the bat. These were people that I had worked with in church, one way or another, but had not really taken the time to get personal with. I had been taught to keep things semi-surfaced to protect myself. This was one of those nifty things Michael had constantly drilled in to me. He had been a victim to being hurt by a church in his past and thus learned to keep his distance from "Church People." He would forever tell me not to get too personal with them; however, distance is one of the things that God said "No more," to.

The first woman who brought us food was a woman I had never taken the time to get to know; I didn't even remember her name. I had directed her husband twice, in two different plays, and by the way,

I had never had a personal conversation with him either. I was very nervous, waiting for her to get here. I did not know what to say or how to act; I did not know where to take the conversation or if I should just excuse myself because I was tired. I was totally consumed and obsessed with my projected scenarios; however, Darling so blessed me when she arrived. Once she walked in, I let go and let God.

As it turned out, she was having similar worries about our encounter but we were able to quickly relax and minister to each other. God can only use a person to the degree to which they are willing to be used. I was completely open to using this situation in any way that God saw fit. If this was my storm, then I wanted to teach people how to sing in the rain. This was how my spirit felt. I was singing in the rain, just singing in the rain, what a glorious feeling, well, you get the idea. I felt that way because God was carrying me; I was tap dancing and singing in the rain. God wanted to inspire those people that He sent to me. It is all right to know that you are inspiring others by your peace, strength, and faith in spite of your circumstances. This is part of our job as Christians: to teach and learn from each other.

Far too many times we give Christianity a bad name because we choose to live like the devil. We walk in fear and not in faith, in hate and not in forgiveness; we walk in despair and not in joy. That is not being responsible for our actions toward each other as Christians. I had earned God's trust by being able to show the positive side of my situation, and in turn, through my example, people were able to see the positive side of whatever they were going through. This is how it is supposed to work. They will know what? They will know we are Christians by our love, our God-given love for one another. I am sure these people had better things to do than spend their time and money on someone who had rarely even bothered to have a conversation with them. God spoke to their hearts and they obeyed.

Staying connected with people who love you is vital to the healing process. There were so many people who wanted to know what was going on with me that I started an e-mail support group. This made it easier for me to update everyone all at once via the computer. Surprisingly, this would prove to be a major support for me throughout the entire healing process. I would encourage anyone who is in the midst of a battle to try this method of communication. I was able to stay connected, even through my times of isolation. The prayer chains that I started through this will be with me for years to come. It also gave me a platform to be able to minister to others. Here is a copy of my first e-mail detailing my condition.

Hey Guys,

Without being cliché, we were so blessed again Friday night by yet a sixth family. It may have taken six days of people bringing us meals to figure it out. It had very little to do with food and last night it came to me. God has been revealing glimpses, just glimpses of the harvest to come through seeds that I have planted. Not through a husband or kids but through seed that I had actually used my own hands to plant. Not many will understand when I say that this is, and has been and continues to be an awesome experience of God's presence in my life. To know that I am on my way and the stagnation is clearing in all areas of my life. I have such an open road ahead of me and I am finally on the right highway. The world would look at my situation and pity me, but I say come on, watch, I am about to take off and fly. I am just getting in some last minute preparations. I will keep you posted on my weekly updates or should I say praise reports as far as health is concerned. I truly thank God for the great times we have shared. But more so for the times yet to come.

I love you guys,
Debbie

God had also shown me how to interact with others. One would be surprised how many people could stand a lesson or two on how to be a friend. Trust me, I am the first in line and looking forward to another class.

The day came for the doctor to remove the bandages and drainage tubes. I had accepted the empty space but I was not ready to actually see it. The doctor removed the bandages so quickly and without warning that I literally threw my hands over my eyes. He said, "What's wrong? It looks good." I said, "Yeah, but can you put the bandages back so I can see it in the privacy of my own home?" He quickly removed the stitches and complied with my wishes. I went back to work and carried on with my daily routine and put it out of my mind.

That evening, after dinner, I went quietly up the stairs to my bedroom and closed the door. I stood in front of the mirror and slowly undressed. When I got to the bandage, I did as the doctor had done and quickly removed it. I was horrified, my breathing was quick and shallow, and I was absolutely stunned. It looked as though I had had my breast ripped off in a horrible car accident and as if they'd tried the best that they could to piece me back together. The area actually sunk in. This looked nothing like the pictures that I'd seen. I thought, how completely cruel not to have warned me.

Then I realized that this was Satan's last attempt to get me to curse my God. I began yelling in the mirror, tears streaming down my cheeks, standing toe to toe with the devil himself. "What? What? What is it that makes you think that I will curse my God? What? What? There is nothing. Nothing! Can't you get that? Nothing! So what if I look like a freak, I will never turn from God again. You are a liar, just leave me alone!" I put both hands on the sink, in my bathroom, dropped my head, and I cried. Actually, I was sobbing and my tears were landing in the sink. I felt that I looked so horrid. I would never want a man to see that. Life without a man was starting to look better and better.

I went downstairs, pulled my mother into the downstairs bathroom, and simply dropped my robe. The horrified look on her face said it all. Although she tried to change her expression quickly, it was too late. This was not a nightmare but my reality. I sat there watching T.V. for an hour with continuous tears streaming down. It was obvious that I was on the verge of a meltdown, and my mom did not know what to expect. The tension was so thick you could cut it with a knife. She just sat there, staring at me. Finally, I popped up and I yelled at her, "What, Mom?! What are you looking at? You want to know why I am crying? You saw what they did to me."

I stormed back upstairs to my room and locked the door. I stood in front of the mirror again, staring at my wound and wondering how much more I could possibly lose. I had been stripped of any and all of my physical beauty that I had been trying to hang on to, and in just a matter of weeks, my beautiful hair would be gone as well. I was melting away into ugliness. I was becoming womanless. I was losing all of my beauty and value as a woman.

Then suddenly, with a roaring voice, God yelled, "Look at me! Look in this mirror! Yes, you are being stripped. Yes, you are losing everything that the world labels as beautiful. However, I am going to show you a beauty which you possess that you would have never discovered otherwise. A beauty that not many women are open enough to find. Then and only then will I restore everything tenfold. You cannot fathom the beauty you're about to step in to, and you are going to show thousands how to find it. They will not have to go this way to get there. You will know the shortcut and remember I love you. With that, I sucked it up, took a shower, and went to bed. When God's message is that clear, how can you argue? I wait with great anticipation for that day of discovery.

My next hurdle would be chemotherapy. I did not waste any time; I started it three weeks after the day of having my mastectomy. When I walked into the infusion center and sat in one of the big recliners, with a sterile smell, I thought to myself, "Man, this just keeps on getting better and better." I was kind of in disbelief that I was actually coming here voluntarily to have them inject medication into my body that was not only going to do good but also do some bad as well. It was all a bit alarming.

The nurse started the IV and then came in with "the stuff." Three large horse-sized syringes filled with drugs. One of them looked like red Kool-Aid. The nurse pulled the curtain closed so that people could not see the tears that once again began rolling down my face. I momentarily started to feel defeated, when just then I remembered that, in anticipation of my long hours of treatment, I had collected a specific list of prayer requests from people at my church, friends, and family. I pulled that list out and started praying like nobody's business. When I started focusing on my problems, I started to sink. No one would blame me, but I was not going to go out like that. I wiped off the tears, opened the curtain, put my hands on the list, and got to work. I had to remember that God was taking care of my stuff and that I should concentrate on helping others. My faith kicked back into high gear, and I was going strong. It was a battle like nothing I had ever faced before, like a tug of war. I would occasionally get pulled back over the line and into the mud, but the power of prayer would get me back onto the land and drag the devil down into the mud, where I would eventually step upon his head and walk out in victory.

The nurse told me that the Kool-Aid-type medication would most likely make my hair fall out within fourteen days but that if I would cut it short, it would do two things: One, I would have a better chance of keeping it because it would be less likely to tangle and pull out through brushing, and two, if it did fall out it would make for an easier transition to go from long hair to short to bald rather than long hair to bald. I had been blessed with big, thick, long, bouncy hair, so bald would be extreme.

So right from the hospital, I went to get my hair cut short. I was going to follow all instructions at this point. I had not had my hair cut short in a very, very long time. I received very different reactions from everyone, from it looking great, to it showing a lack of faith in what God could do, to I should not have done it until I had to. I had to believe that God was guiding my every step and dismiss anything remotely negative. I had to realize that not many would truly understand the effects and impact of this particular storm on my life and the lives of my children. I really had to conserve energy and pick my battles wisely.

Three hours after leaving the hospital, I was sick. I did not see the light of day for four days except for the two rides to the hospital to get intravenous fluids. I could not even keep down a sip of water. Suddenly, the mastectomy looked like a cakewalk. The most depressing thing was that this was only the beginning; I had months to go. I slept for hours on end, I lost track of the world, I slept to get away, and I had discovered a new depth of loneliness.

22

Now I Felt Blinded
by the Battle

At this point in my life, it's fair to say that the effects of the chemo were surely in control. I could physically feel my flesh and the effects of the treatment going at it, battling head to head, and I was definitely cheering for my flesh. I was trying to help my body as much as I could, so I would give myself positive pep talks and try to push the fluids. I valiantly fought off the negativity to not feed the cancer that was under attack. By the fifth day, I emerged from my room the victor. Although I was weak and beaten up, still I was the victor all the same. As I started to regain my strength, I found that I so appreciated feeling good. Here is the e-mail update I sent out to my support group.

Hey Guys,
What can I say? I was knocked out for a minute with my first chemo treatment. I had not properly prepared mentally. Sitting in that chair for 3 hours while they physically push toxins into your body is, is, I cannot even find the words at the moment. I will admit that I shed quite a few tears as I almost fell into a pity party for myself but I quickly remembered the prayer requests, got my notes, and started warring. I would periodically fall back on myself but for the most part, intercessory prayer was my best weapon. Thank you for the ammunition. Please feel free to send others if a need arises. Yes, I cut my hair. I was told that I would have a better chance of keeping it if it were short. Your hair gets dry and brittle, which makes

it tangle and fall out more the longer your hair is. I was also told that they found "something" on one of my ovaries and that I would need further testing. When I say that I was knocked out, I mean nausea and vomiting within 3 hours of leaving the hospital. I could not even keep down a sip of water. I had to go in to the hospital twice for dehydration and it took four days to pass. The awesome thing was that it did pass. I can deal with down four days because that means I get 2 weeks and three days that are great. Wednesday was my fifth day and I had to go in for the ultrasound on my ovaries, which was a bit intrusive, if I do say so myself. While I was lying there in this dark room, being probed, I thought, "What else?" Ovarian cancer? Fine! Pull it all out! I am done having kids anyway. All the tech said was, "Oh, there it is." When I asked her what, she just told me that I would have to speak to my doctor. So, on my way home I felt as if I was losing my footing. I just kept saying fine, do whatever needs to be done.

I pulled over, reached for my cell phone, and called the church administrator and said, a bit incoherently, "Have you ever felt as if the devil was so pissed that you keep on getting up that he has to pull out all the stops and come at you with everything that he's got?" Needless to say, if you were at church on Wednesday night, you heard God's response to me. I will never face this giant again. God also told me that it all has to be discovered so that it can all be dealt with at one time. You prayed for a complete healing so I must bring it out to the surface to be dealt with. Relax! I have it all under control. Just making it to praise and worship had my spirit soaring. I was told not to be around a lot of people or crowds but I so need to be at service. So, if I come and go without notice, it is just that I need to stay clear of crowds and germs. Keep the drama dept. in prayer. We start on Tuesday. Please let me know if you need anything. I truly love you all and your support is thrilling. Please do not hesitate to share your thoughts with me.

God Bless You!

Debbie

It was now Easter Sunday and I was at a barbecue at a friend's house. There was a gentle, cool breeze blowing as we all sat outside with our plates piled with food. Let's just say that I gave new meaning to the phrase, "My hair was blowing in the wind." At first people were noticing a hair here and a hair there, then it got worse, and suddenly I realized that it was coming from my head. I quickly put my hands over my head in an effort to stop the hair from flying. A friend then gave me a scarf to tie on my head. I didn't know whether to laugh or cry; I noticed that everyone was waiting for my reaction, which I knew would determine how they would react, so I decided to make light of the situation, which in turn put everyone else at ease. So, when I got home I ran a brush through my hair just once, it was full of hair, I mean completely full of my once-beautiful hair; it gave me chills. This continued for two days; I was shedding like a dog, literally. My kids kept trying to pick all the extra hair that had fallen onto my shoulders and back.

Hey guys,
The awesome news is: no ovarian cancer. It is just a cyst. I am getting ready for round number two of chemo. I think this time I will be ready for the punch. Unfortunately, I was not the one out of ten to keep their hair. It started falling out two days ago. I must say it is a bit of a drag. The last thing you want to do is see people. It is very embarrassing and definitely drains the mind. Tonight I was blessed with a night of praise and worship at church, which always puts my soul at peace. Have a blessed weekend.
Love
Debbie

Despite my best efforts, my hair loss was affecting everyone who saw me. Pastor Linda at church saw that it was obvious that I would soon be bald and was a bit shaken. She announced that the women of the church were going to throw me a hat party due to my inevitable hair loss. I had never before experienced such a show of support by people who were not related to me. God was just showering me every step of the way. God was saturating me, through people. These were people I had seen for years but never met. I was given more hats, scarves, and earrings than I knew what to do with. My illness was being used to pull the women of the church together like never before. I knew that this was a new beginning for us all as women with pains. We gained the courage to reach out to one another and it felt right; it felt strong. I knew it was the start of something powerful; we were free to care for each other. I felt God's strength! Don't get me wrong; I was shocked at my hair falling out by the handfuls, but never did it devastate me. However, it did seem to affect some of the women even more than it affected me because they were envisioning how they would have reacted if it had happened to them and how terribly bad they felt for me. I was back to comforting them and reassuring them that it was going to be all right. I started to look like a Charlie Brown character with just a few straggling hairs. Finally I called my friend Monica because she was a hair stylist. She opened up her shop when it was closed and she quietly shaved my head for me in private. Sometimes it is just easier to embrace the inevitable. Thank you Monica.

From that day on, every time I went to church, I was given a gift of some kind. Earrings, scarves, picture frames, and turbans. One service, a couple simply placed a check for $1,000.00 in my hand and whispered in my ear, "Be blessed," and then embraced me! Talk about being at a loss for words. I always seemed to be crying at church but it was not from sorrow, it was from complete joy. I then started to realize that no man had ever made me feel as loved and complete as God had throughout my ordeal. That is because I had never stayed put long enough for God to show Himself to me in my life. I had always let something or someone draw my attention away from Him. This time I was not going anywhere until I knew for sure that it was God leading me. So on with chemo treatment number three.

Hi Guys,

Yes, three down and seven to go. Because my body was handling the negative effects of the chemotherapy so well and my strength was holding up, the doctor decided to go ahead with the maximum number of treatments from six to ten. The down side of course is obvious, the up side is that I will be less likely to face cancer ever again. This is definitely a half full situation. I am doing well tonight. I am in the best place in my life because I have learned to look to God to fulfill my needs. The added blessing is that he chooses to use people like you to love me through. There is not a day that goes by that one of you reach out to my spirit. Whether it be through encouragement, giving, joining me in battle, or even giving me the opportunity to help you. It always comes at the perfect time. Right when I start to teeter, someone catches me. Just when I start to feel like a joke or like, what is the point, God lets me know the point through one of you. If you are having trouble in the midst of your storm, let me help you. I was going to say follow me, but that is not the answer. Follow God! Now, if God

uses others in the process, that will work but ultimately God is waiting on you to rely on HIM! For the first time in my life, there is no middle man. When it comes time to stand before God, I can guarantee that it will be you and you alone.
I Love You & Many Blessings
Debbie

I had always had good skin and a great complexion. I now had dry, blotchy skin that was peeling with dark patches. I was losing my eyebrows and my eyelashes but at this point, it all seemed irrelevant to what was really going on. God had finally received my full and complete attention.

23

God Continued Bringing Reinforcements

We had a guest speaker at our church; his name is E. Vann Walker. He called me up to the pulpit during the service and proceeded to pray for healing and speak over my life. He said, "God spoke to me about you while I was preaching; you will not die a premature death. I speak to the death angel: You have to leave right now. Debbie, this sickness is not unto death but unto the glory of God." He then turned and addressed the congregation: "You know, this woman is not even supposed to be alive right now." And then he came right back to me, "Literally, you are living resurrection life. You're not even supposed to be alive. You're only alive because God has purpose for your life and because the King has the last word. If infirmities had the last word, sweetheart, you would have been gone already. But the King, the King has the last word. And by the time God gets done with you, you are going to be one of the devil's worst nightmares. And guess what, everything you lost, you're going to get it all back. And the King appointed someone to get it all back and she recovered all. You are not a sick woman. I don't want you to live like a sick woman. I don't want you to act like a sick woman. I don't want you to praise like a sick woman. I want you to continue to function like you are alive and well, because guess what? You are. And when the devil puts a period on something, the thing I love about God is that God will come and put a comma on a period."

As you can imagine, I was on cloud nine. I was smiling from ear to ear. I did not even move from the sanctuary for at least thirty minutes after the service was over. The church was empty, eighty percent of the lights were out, and I was still beaming with joy; it is somewhat easy to be beaming with joy when you have 400 people and a man of God behind you.

When I woke up the next morning, I was still walking on air. I got up, went to work, and worked my first full day in six months. I had added many special projects on my plate. I went to three different gatherings, which included a wedding and reception, and by the end of the week, I was sick. It started as the flu, then went on to bronchitis, and when you throw a dose of chemo in there, you land in bed for over a month. Now this did not exactly line up with what I thought my prophecy said. Or maybe I'd just heard what I wanted to hear. Let us go back, shall we? E. Vann Walker had said, "I want you to CONTINUE to function like you are alive and well." Continue! He did not say add or increase, he merely said continue. This meant what I was doing was working. I was on the right track and somehow took a detour, which landed me on a tougher road for a moment. Let me rephrase that: a much, much tougher road for quite a few moments. I could not sleep lying down; I had fever, sweats, sore throat, cracked lips, sores in my mouth, stomachaches, headaches; you name it, I had it. I could not get out of bed for my daughter's twelfth birthday, and I was not able to even think of getting her a present or a cake. I was so mad at myself.

And just to add a little salt to the wound, she went to dinner with her dad and his girlfriend as well as his family. You can only imagine what a blow that was to my mommy ego. I simply gave her a kiss as she left to celebrate without me. I somehow mustered enough strength though to have a little pity party all by myself, in my room, in the dark with lots and lots of tears. But when my daughter came home loaded with presents, with a beaming smile all I could say was, "Thank you, Lord, for blessing my daughter, thank you for not missing her special day, and thank you for having my back."

That night as I lay there in the dark, I was reminded of that song that says, "Late in the midnight hour, God's going to turn it around. It's gonna work in your favor." Well, this was as good a night as any, so start turning. Then I thought about how I felt at that service when I'd received that prophecy, how I was walking on cloud nine. Then the Holy Spirit said, "It's easy to believe when you have four hundred people behind you, it is easy to believe when a man of God calls you out, and it is easy to ride on the faith of others. Now, can you believe by yourself? Can you recognize me in the dark? Do you know my touch?" I took a moment ...

I began to feel hot on the inside and then it turned into a calming warmth. I felt my smile start to get bigger and bigger, as I realized Yes! I sat up in my bed with excitement and said, "Yes, despite what it looked like, I do believe. It is my faith. I believe." I had been isolated for a month, and I still believed. It is not a feeling, an emotion, or getting caught up in the hype of it all; my faith is real and it is all mine. I love God and want nothing but His will in my life. I started to cry with tears of absolute joy because God gave me proof that night that my heart and beliefs were real, just as real as my pillow and my blanket. Just as real as anything that I could put my hands on. That night, I experienced a true revelation, and no one will ever be able to take that away from me. No one! So now I will just continue.

4 Down, 6 To Go

Hey Guys,
Sorry it has been awhile. This last chemo was a slam to my system. Looking back, I let my guard down and made some bad decisions in participating in some group activities when I was feeling ill. Being fragile is a new world to me. I must say I do not remember ever being that sick for that long before. The Lord is really teaching me about doing what is right for me. I cannot afford any more mistakes. A person can be devoured in those dark, lonely, and depressing places that one finds themselves in, in sickness. And yes, for a minute or two or even three, I felt completely alone, and then I remembered all that God has promised me and I knew I was and am never alone. Knowing that, is all I had to keep in mind. Man, this is no game. I can usually just plow my way through most obstacles but this is such a long and consistently draining process, one tends to lose sight of the light at the end of the tunnel. Then I look around and see my family being drained as well. My kids are showing signs of not knowing what the future holds, worrying if they will lose their mom as well. When I disappeared to my room for a week, I saw insecurity start to rise. When I could not even come out for Cheyenne's birthday, they knew it was serious. I pray that whatever

God is trying to show those around me that it gets through. I am trying my hardest not to miss a thing and I encourage those around me to do the same. Let's get the most out of all of this, together. Let's watch God turn around what the devil meant for evil. I was told that when God is done with all of this that I would be the devil's worst nightmare. That sounds awesome to me. In this past crisis, there were extremely blessed gestures by family and friends. But I must say, Lucy, Michele, & Billy, I love you guys. You consistently leave me without words. Thanks for loving my girls. You step in just when I think I have let my girls down. I thank God for bringing you into our lives. I still say that I am in the best place in my life because finally my life is in God's hands.
God Bless,
Debbie

Everything was telling me to focus on the next treatment, to get ready, be healthy, concentrate on getting to the halfway point and do not get thrown by anything. I felt as if I was playing dodge ball and I just kept getting hit. I was definitely frustrated but I was not going to be beaten. I remember thinking how unfair it was that I was alone, meaning without a significant other by my side. I had no one to hold me, no one longing to hear my voice, much less see my face or wonder what I was doing.

It would have been easy to get lost in those thoughts, so I would just bury them. I was certain that I was not going to get involved with anyone until my divorce was final, which was a whole different nightmare in itself. As far as I was concerned, I was still a married woman, and this time, I would act accordingly. After my first divorce, I got married three days later. Obviously, I did not wait until I was available. Like I'd said before, I did to my first husband what basically was done to me by Michael. Perhaps that has a lot to do with me not lashing back at Michael and his girlfriend. I am far from being an angel or a saint. The fact of the matter was that I had been there and I had done that literally. You can call it karma, what goes around comes around, or whatever you want; the point is I fought very hard not to put myself above anyone, including Michael and his girlfriend.

For the past two years, I lived in hiding. Remember, Michael and his girlfriend lived in the same condominium complex and worked together in the same shopping center as I did. Their presence had become a stronghold in my life, and I allowed it to hold me prisoner. It had ruled and dictated my every move. Originally, I hid out to protect myself from humiliation as well as heartbreak because I was devastated and still in love. What ended up happening was that I was so distracted by their presence that I even missed when my heart had been healed; I missed when the love was gone.

Trust me when I say, "Do not let yourself be that distracted by anything." You will absolutely want to recognize when a healing of this magnitude occurs in your life. A person's true freedom depends on acknowledging it. I remember that day of realization: The two of them had come by to pick my girls up for a visit. I was sitting in the living room looking very bad with no make-up and wearing dumpy clothes. I was suffering the effects of my latest chemo treatment, and I was getting up to vomit in the bathroom when I heard the horn honking. I walked into the bathroom and looked at my reflection in the mirror. While I was leaning on the counter, trying to decide if I was going to throw up or not, I simply said, "No more." I was tired of the prison that I had put myself in, so I walked out of the bathroom, opened the front door, and went outside. I remember my older daughter violently grabbing me by the arm and saying, "Where are you going?" She had a very distressed look on her face, so to comfort her, I looked at her, smiled, and said, "Don't worry, baby girl."

I was on a mission; I was finally going to bust out of that prison. I approached their car with a smile and warm greeting. I kindly said that my girls would be out in a moment. The very next moment, my girls came out to get in their car, and when my older daughter hugged me, she whispered in my ear, "You are so brave, Mom. I am so proud of you."

I cannot tell you what my husband and his girlfriend were thinking but they did appear to be a bit shocked and at a loss for words but then again I did look like a poster child for cancer.

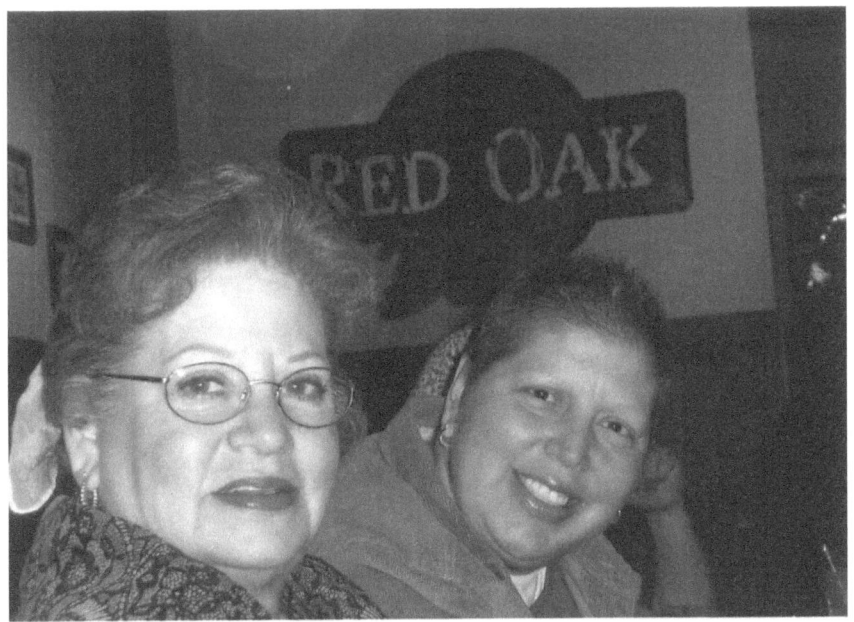

A picture of me with little hair

With that simple gesture, I was free. My children and I were free. I had unknowingly taken them into that prison right along with me. Do not get me wrong: When I got back into the house, my own shock set in: the realization of him picking her over me, her looking all cute, and I was looking as bad as I ever had in my entire life and having to face it as well as accepting it all.

24

What's It Going to Take?

Believe it or not, after two years, Michael had still not filed the proper paperwork for our divorce; however, my daughters told me that he had already given his girlfriend an engagement ring. His audacity and flagrant disregard for completing our divorce was unnerving. Obviously, I would never take him back, so it was not about the heartbreak; as a matter of fact, part of me felt as though she was getting exactly what she deserved. Someone once told me that when a woman steals another woman's husband, the best revenge is to let her keep him. I did, however, feel yet again that life was being a bit unfair. He seemed to have his new life well under way, while I felt that I was stuck in a reaping mode.

The thing about envy is that things are never what they seem; the grass is not always greener on the other side. In reality, I would not trade places with either one of them. Another thing that I have come to realize is that when a person is right in the middle of their storm, which is exactly where I was, their storm appears to be much worse than those around them. This is simply not true; one never truly knows what others are facing. I had to stop looking at everybody else and focus on what was in front of me.

So, yes, I would still have ill thoughts from time to time but just as quickly as they came, I was able to release them. I prayed for the release of any and all strongholds in my life. I examined my life as well as my choices, which in turn revealed and gave me names to those strongholds. It is important for you to know what your strongholds are so that you can physically and verbally speak to them in order to release them. If you do not know what they are, you will not be able to release them. It is like cleaning out a closet; unless you reach in and grab the junk, you'll never be able to throw it away, and once you start cleaning, you will most likely find some garbage in there that you either forgot about or did not even know you had. The added benefit of cleaning out your closet is that you make more room for the things of God.

5 Down, 5 To Go

Hello,
Does it seem as though I am getting anywhere? This past Thursday I had surgery to install a chemo port due to the fact that my veins are shot. Friday I found out it was unsuccessful. Friday I had chemo and all went well. I did get sick but it is normal chemo sickness. No flu or bronchitis, which is a very good thing. I am still very weak which is very annoying but I am still moving forward. I miss you all. You do not realize how much you are all a part of my backup troops. God is just so awesome to me. Keep up the good work.
God Bless,
Debbie

So there you have it, I'd made it halfway through; the operative word being "through." It seemed as though the halfway point in my chemotherapy was going to be a bigger accomplishment than it actually was because all it meant was that I still had the same amount of grief coming all over again. With each treatment, I was getting a little closer to death. What I mean is, each treatment killed the bad stuff as well as the good stuff. That's the tradeoff for the cure, or should I say, life. I knew I was not actually going to die but I knew that I would get close enough to be able to look death right in the face, eye to eye. Then I would smile and tell him goodbye, turn, and work my way back to a new life.

I will never see things the same way again, and that is an awesome thing. I was already living a different life; I had such an appreciation for people. I could even appreciate people that I had never met.

I have a cousin who lives in Chicago, and he works for Chanel. That year I decided to commemorate the halfway mark of my treatment and my forty-fourth birthday at the same time with a family picture, which would obviously mark my baldness as well. Once I received the photograph, I sent the picture to all of my e-mail prayer partners, including him.

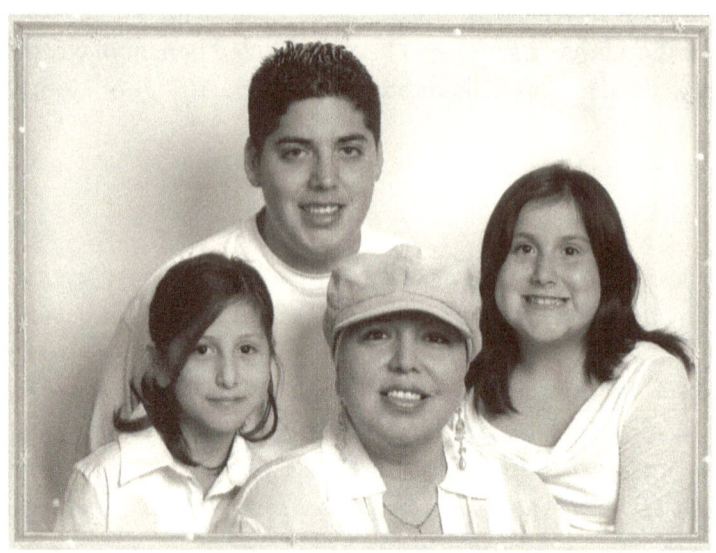

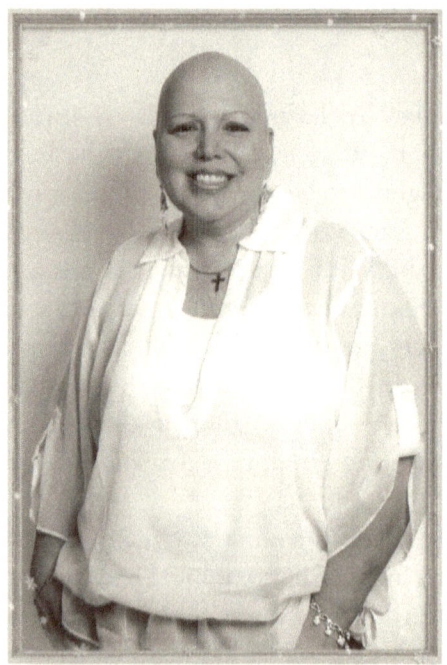

He must have shared my picture as well as my story with some of his co-workers, because I received a Fed-Ex package from his office. In the package was a card signed by about twenty people I had never met nor spoken to, and whom, might I add, worked for Chanel as well.

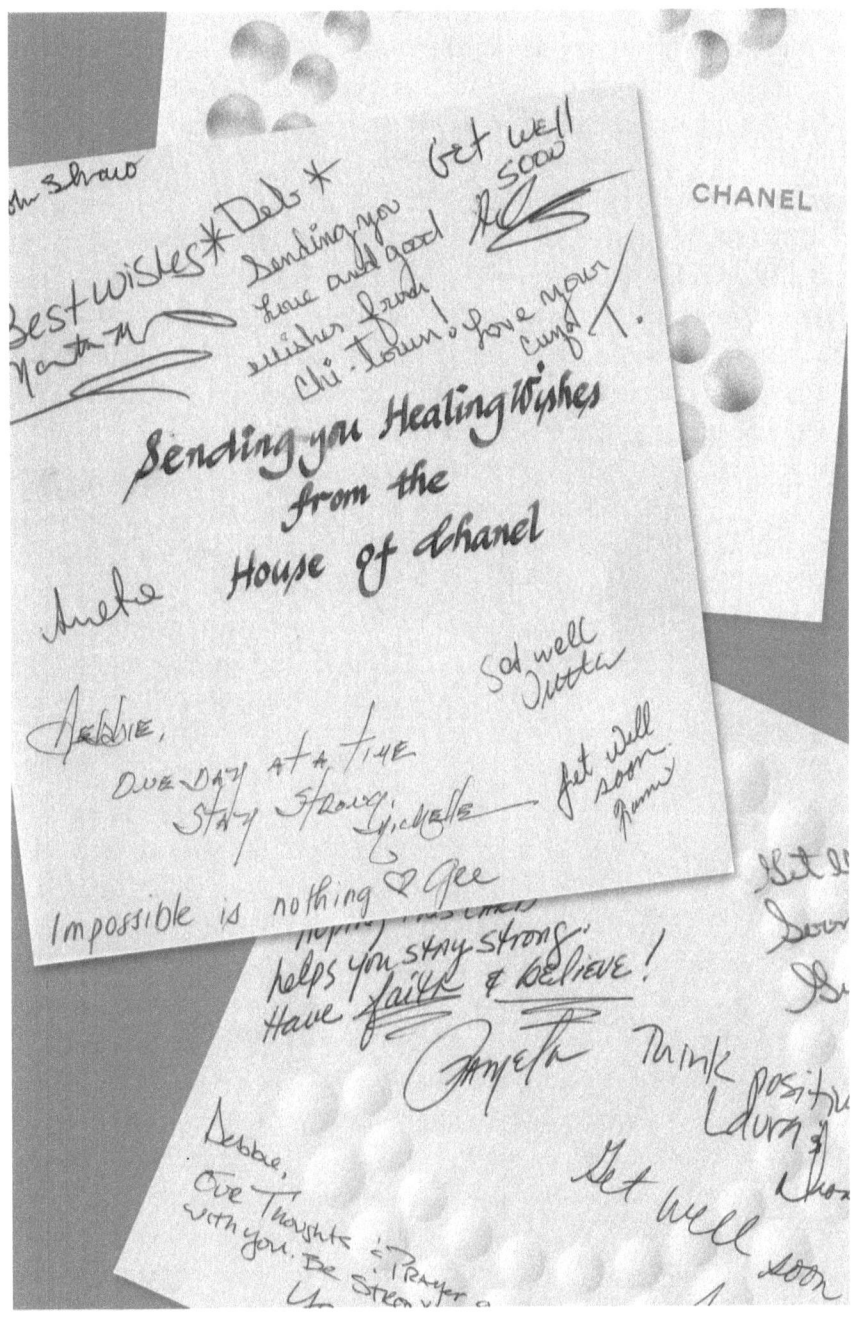

There was also a small black box with a white Chanel ribbon. I opened the box to find a beautiful pair of diamond earrings inside. I found myself, once again, speechless and in tears. God was reaching clear across the United States, to people I had never even met, in order to bless me. The earrings looked too beautiful to put on, so I just kept peeking in the box every so often. This was on a Friday. I finally decided that I would wear them on Sunday when I went to church. Hey, if God was blessing, then I was dressing. Never underestimate the power of giving to those who are in a battle. Just allow God to flow through you and follow God's lead to give to others. Although those people at Chanel never knew the impact that their gift had in my healing process, I am a witness to the power of kindness. Take it from someone whose life has been transformed by the kindness of others, not to mention the blessings that come to those who have been obedient to what God has asked of them. For me, it was not about being materialistic. You see, I could not bring myself to even try the earrings on because at that point in my life, I didn't feel pretty enough nor worthy of wearing something so beautiful. It is about feeling that you are valuable and precious, about realizing that you are special to God, and He spares no expense. He uses any and all means to let you know what you mean to Him. And there, my friends, is a prime example of God's will in your life.

6 Down, 4 To Go

Hey Guys
The numbers are getting to be more in my favor. I feel great and strong in the midst of weakness. Hey! Is that what it means, "When I am weak, He is strong." WOW! How awesome is that? I am over the hump. By September, we are finished with this course. I say we because God gave me all of you to help me through, and I must say that you have done a tremendous job. Please keep in mind that we are not over the finish line yet. I know that I have been out of sight but please do not let my children and I leave your minds. Never underestimate your part in the victories of those you pray for. Your prayers help hold my arms up when I can no longer do it myself. Satan would love me to believe that I am alone in this battle, late at night, in the dark, with tears slowly getting lost in my pillow. But I know that that is the lie and that I am far from being alone. Thank you for being with me and my children in our darkest of nights.

God Bless.
Debbie

I felt as if I was gaining some ground; six down, four to go. The first series was over. My next treatment would be a new drug, which leaves room for better reaction to treatment. However, when I read the side effects, I wondered, how is that possible and when would it get better? I might lose my nails on both my fingers and toes, I might swell up like the Pillsbury doughboy and a host of other nifty side dishes, but I could not focus on that; my focus had to be on the fact that I only had four treatments left. I was planning a trip to Hawaii the next summer with family and friends. I also had planned to go to New York the following Christmas. I was going to live and love and laugh and be the best I could be with this new chance at life.

The Fourth of July was two days away, and I was feeling pretty good, so I decided to throw a barbecue at my house. I wanted to bless a few of the people who had been helping me get through the past two years; I just wanted them to walk in and be blessed. It was an awesome day; that one day, everyone in my house was blessed and experienced joy because of God's efforts, through me. Recognize that no matter where you are, in the midst or fully out of a storm, God will always use a willing heart.

The highlight was when some unexpected guests showed up from San Francisco. They brought a beautiful sunflower bouquet for me, as evidence that the Lord still reaches out in many directions to bless me, from the earrings from Chicago to the beautiful bouquet all the way from San Francisco to my home in Whittier, I am blessed. When I saw my surprise visitors and the flowers at my doorstep, tears of elation just came down. I thank God for allowing me to recognize Him in my life every day, through the good days as well as the rough ones. Remember what the Bible says: "He will never leave you nor forsake you."

7 Down and Only 3 Left

Now that's what I'm talking about. All of a sudden, the end feels near. I started on a new drug and I seem to be taking it well. I had it on Thursday and went to work today. This treatment took twice as long but I do not care because I do not feel nauseated. Blessed be the name of the Lord, Amen. I can see the light at the end of the tunnel. Yes, it's still a bit away but hey, I

CAN SEE IT!!! I CAN FEEL IT!!! I CAN TASTE IT!!!
I THINK YOU GET THE POINT. AND YES, I AM YELLING!!!!! I
recently met a woman whom I have had a correspondence with but have never
met. We are walking the exact same walk, we are literally at the same place
in treatment. I was recently given the honor of meeting her in person over an
awesome dinner. It was like meeting a soul survivor, we knew without words.
Lord, you are just too much for words. Vivian, you are truly a blessing in my life
and are an awesome and mighty woman of God. In ten days from now, Vivian
and I shall be bald again but hey, we have learned how to make it look good.
Please add Vivian to your prayer list. We need all the prayers we can get.
God Bless,
Debbie

Maybe I was counting my eggs before they hatched. This time it took a few days for the lightning to strike. And strike it did. This brief moment of rest was all I had before another wage of war began.

Side Effects

O.K. Yes, the side effects started to show up with a vengeance on Monday morning. It started with full body aches and cramping. My mouth is completely filled with mouth sores and thrush, which makes eating a very bad experience. I have silver dollar-size sores on my hands and feet which affects my walking, sitting, and using my hands, I have a rash on my head, which makes lying down an issue, and as of yesterday, my white blood cells are shot, they are simply gone. If I do not want to be hospitalized, I must stay home, away from people, which means no visitors until I can build up some kind of defense, maybe by next week. They have determined that the dosage of the new drug was too strong, so next time they will lower it. Just when you think you cannot go any further, the morning comes and you start again. Even if you have to drag yourself up, the point is that you are up. I am always amazed at how God is always a step ahead of me. Please keep my children and my Mom and Dad in prayer. I can see their weariness. I can only pray that they are learning from watching me. They see me cry in pain and distress but I work through, I do not stop. I know it hurts them to see me. I would love to send them away so they would not have to watch but I get to a point of helplessness and I physically need them to help me. I know it looks like I am being beaten but my flesh is what they are seeing and I need them to see and know that my spirit soars. If anything, that is what I pray you

all can witness. It would be a shame for any of you to miss that.
Be blessed,
Debbie

25

My Children Were Wearing Thin

My elder daughter began showing signs of major stress; she was consumed by fears and worries; she could not eat and was rapidly losing weight. She was watching me as my symptoms worsened and was worried sick that her mother was going to die. She told me that if I died, she wanted to die with me. She began worrying about her future and about her dad, and she was experiencing intense growing pains in her legs that often brought her to tears, and if all that weren't enough, she was just around the corner from becoming a little lady. I made an appointment and took her to see the doctor just as soon as I could pull it together.

Thankfully, there was nothing medically wrong with her but the doctor suspected early signs of an eating disorder and suggested counseling. My daughter was desperate for help. It seemed as though everywhere we went, she was looking for help. She spoke to our pastor, a priest, and a couple of women leaders from our church as well as our family counselor. She was so fearful that she suspected a demonic presence in our home, and she asked a couple from our church to come pray over our house and bless it with oil. Her sense of security was being threatened. Truth be told, these children had been dragged through the mud right along with me. Even my son and younger daughter were showing signs of wear and tear in their own ways.

Therefore, I started praying right along with my e-mail group as well as focusing on the problems at hand. Within two hours of requesting prayer for my family, my children were blessed with a full social schedule to help take their minds off our obvious circumstances. On Thursday, Cheyenne was invited to an all-day beach party. Friday, all three kids were taken to Universal Studios. Saturday, the girls went to an eighties birthday party, with one of them winning first prize for her Madonna costume. Sunday, all four of us were taken to Ringling Brothers and Barnum & Bailey Circus.

In addition, on the following Wednesday, my girls were taken to the happiest place on Earth, Disneyland. Keep in mind, I did not pay a penny for any of these excursions. We were completely blessed by friends and family as well as complete strangers. It was as simple as God stepping in, taking our focus off the bad, and getting us back into life. Within two hours, God moved on that many people and by the end of seven days, we were smiling and joyous again. When a person is being whipped around in a storm, it is very easy to lose focus. Even though I was the captain of my ship, I was dropping the sail here and there, which in turn threw us way off course. Because of the fact that I was willing to reach out for help and readjust, getting back on track came very easily. I let God take the helm and followed directions, and in seven days, we were back on track. There was still quite a mess to clean up, mind you, but the damage was contained and dealt with.

Praise Report

Good Morning,

I hope you are well today. Here is my praise report. The side effects started to subside yesterday. Little by little, things are returning to normal. My mouth is almost clear. I am starting to have taste. The rash on my head is gone. The sores on my hands and feet are starting to shrink. Last, but not least, the heaviness has lifted. I know I keep saying it but man, this is draining stuff. I feel like I'm in a boxing match and I only get 60 seconds between rounds to catch my breath. I start envisioning Rocky Balboa and how hopeless it looked toward the end as he stammered about, not to mention how he looked. The exciting part is we all know how it ends. I know how this will end. I know that this victory is going to be as exciting as Rocky Balboa getting that knockout. Three rounds left. Do not get up and go to the bathroom now or you will miss the knockout of the year. I love you,

Debbie
P.S. We need my white blood cells to make a complete recovery. I go in on Thursday to have them checked.

I was no longer in pain, but as the sores dried up on my hands and feet, the skin began to crack and peel; it was gross. The dry skin was just coming off in big pieces. It looked most unattractive and felt even worse, scratchy and rough. I was starting to really appreciate the fact that I had no significant man in my life. I didn't have to try to figure out if he was losing interest in me or not.

Michael happened to ask me if I thought he would have been able to handle my sickness if we had still been together; I asked myself that same question, and the answer was, absolutely not. What was he talking about? He lost interest in me when I was well; how could he possibly think that he could have handled this? Moreover, how could he even ask me that question?

I was feeling as though I was at the most unattractive place in my life, and to add misery to pain, it did not help that Michael's girlfriend was about sixteen years younger than I was. She was cute, petite, and young. How in the world was I supposed to compete with that? The point is, I was not supposed to be competing, period. Therefore, God stepped in and cleared all that mess out of my life beforehand. God knew what was coming my way. It was like fixing a caved-in roof in summer and not trying to deal with it in the middle of El Niño. If the roof had not been replaced, there is a good possibility that I would have died in the storm I was in with cancer.

It had always been in my nature to put Michael first. I remember the birth of our first daughter. She was twelve pounds, and yes, ladies and gentlemen, I had her naturally. That is only because by the time the doctor realized how big she was, her head was already crowning. When I saw my knees go past my ears, I knew that I was in trouble. I still do not know how she came out. I think I tried to block it out but what I do remember is that in the midst of trying to push her out, what I was really worried about more was if my husband was O.K. I remember, just moments before giving birth, through the toughest part of my labor, I was apologizing to him for crying in pain. This is just another example of how little I thought of myself and how much

I thought of him. God was clearing all of that out so that I would have the ability to be able to concentrate on myself. Taking care of me first was new to me, and taking care of me first for my children's sake was a concept that I actually loved and felt right about.

I cannot go back and reclaim the sixteen years that I had squandered on someone who was unworthy. I can only learn from the past and cherish my future. I implore anyone reading this story to learn the value of who you are, learn the value of your God-given talents, and learn what pearls you hold; never throw them to the swine but use them to further the kingdom of God. You may think this sounds a bit harsh but that is exactly what the Bible says:

Matthew 7:6: Do not give dogs what is sacred; do not throw your pearls to pigs, If you do, they may trample them under their feet, and then turn and tear you to pieces.

"Turn and tear you to pieces." I have stood on both sides of this scripture, I have been the swine and I have been torn to pieces. The point of the scripture is to stay clear of both sides and to protect your God-given pearls so they can be used for their God-given purpose. I have spent most of my life picking and choosing things from the Bible. I ignored the parts that would condemn or chastise my life style, and I used what worked to support my desires. That is not how it is supposed to work; we do not get to pick and choose, dissecting what we like and dislike. The Bible is a manual for life, complete and in its entirety.

How many times have you gotten something new and rather than reading the instructions, you try to figure it out on your own, having to work twice as hard by going back and starting over again when you got it wrong? What is it that makes us think that we know it all and that we can figure out our lives on our own?

That is exactly what we are doing by not knowing God's word. Until a person takes responsibility for reading and knowing God's word, we will always come up short. You end up living a life filled with turmoil and strife, not knowing the strategy to be victorious. Understand that there is a definite difference between turmoil and strife, as opposed to trials and storms. Turmoil and strife are brought on by bad decisions, while trials and storms are there for us to overcome and learn valuable lessons from. I do not recall "live a life of lawlessness" as being one of the Ten Commandments.

Matthew 7:23: Then I will tell them plainly, "I never knew you; Away from Me, you evildoers!"

Yet, this was the kind of life I'd ended up living. Remember this: Whenever you're thinking that the momentary pleasure is worth the pain of the consequence, turn and run in the other direction. To say you will be sorry ends up being a very, very big understatement because you never know the true price of something until after you've bought it, and remember, you will reap what you sow.

Galatians 6:7-8: Do not be deceived, God cannot be mocked; A man reaps what he sows. The one who sows to please his sinful nature, from that nature will reap destruction; the one who sows to please the spirit, from the Spirit will reap eternal life.

The awesome thing about figuring out that you're off-track is that all you have to do is reposition yourself. God's grace will cover the rest!

James 4:6-7: But He gives more grace. That is why scripture says: "God opposes the proud but gives grace to the humble." Submit yourselves, then, to God. Resist the devil and he will flee from you.

It does not get any clearer than that. The problem is, if you never read the manual, the Bible, the directions, how can you know what to do? The first part of my life, the first forty years, is a perfect example of that, but just watch the second half. It is going to be phenomenal. I am off to an outstanding start, if I do say so myself. So on we go with the battle.

26

I Needed to See Myself Through God's Eyes

I tried to take advantage of the days that I felt O.K. One particular Saturday, I was feeling good so I decided to run some errands. I was getting a lot done, and I will go so far as to say that on this day I felt beautiful and strong. I had pep in my step and a smile for everyone I ran into. For the first time since cancer hit, I had forgotten my circumstances. Everything from my husband living one block over with the other woman, my baldness, my absence of color from nine months of no sun, to missing one breast. I somehow, if only for a moment, had forgotten what I looked like, which was a poster child for cancer.

Then, I walked past a mirror and instantaneously, it all came back to me like a flood. I saw my stature immediately drop as soon as I saw my reflection in the mirror. I felt my facial muscles slowly slip downward. I said to myself, "Oh, there you are. I had forgotten about you." As I stood there in tears and in shock at how quickly my mood had shifted, God said, "What you were walking in was your true beauty, you were walking in what I see when I look at you, we were walking together. You were walking in what people can see IN you. What you are looking at now standing before you in front of this mirror is merely flesh. Your flesh is what has kept you from seeing your true self within, which is where I dwell. Now that what you'd perceived as beauty, which was only outer beauty, has been stripped and is gone, only now you are able to experience the true beauty which, through all of this heartbreak and disease, is now developing because of the choices you are now making to draw near to Me. It could not have been restored because you'd never made the choices that would've allowed this type of inner beauty to develop. In your fight to subdue your flesh, your spirit has evolved. One does not look at a butterfly and say that it has returned to its true beauty; its beauty has come through by remaining in its cocoon long enough to become a thing of beauty."

I had made it. I'd stayed in my cocoon long enough to become a thing of beauty from within. In that moment of realization, I fell in love with God. I felt warm, safe, content, secure, wanted, and adored by God.

God told me that I had entered into a special place that not many people ever get to because they either break out of their cocoon too early or are ripped out by the people in their lives or by circumstances that cause them to quit before they are done. A true thing of beauty, to be gracious, giving, loving, and an uplifting person, takes a lot of work and time. It is far easier to be self-centered, selfish, condemning, self-serving, and negative.

I have become a person that people truly love, enjoy, respect, admire, and genuinely like to be around. I live to inspire and guide others through their storms by example and not just in word. "Do as I do" is my new mantra; my actions speak for themselves. Is that conceited? Absolutely not, because this is what comes from embracing the characteristics of Christ. Life is not just about making a way for oneself, it's about making it through as a body all together and many as one, because we were created to need and love one another.

As a believer in Christ, I embrace being a part of the human race and strive on a daily basis to do my part for our betterment. I know that my children are learning by my example. I have finally reached the place where I can say that I want them to learn from me, because now I know that I am worth learning from. I finally see myself as worthy, and I know that I can make it because of Christ, who lives in me. Once a person knows their worth, they will know their value, and in knowing their value, they will see the reason to keep forging ahead.

Hey Guys,
I cannot tell how many times I have seen the finish line in life but have never

made it across. In each battle, I find the part you are in is most important. First, you must start, then fight, then finish and rejoice in your victory. Hebrews 12:1: "Therefore we also, since we are surrounded by so great a cloud of witnesses, let us lay aside every weight, and the sin which so easily ensnares us, and let us run with endurance the race that is set before us." We are all in some battle. Let's all meet over the finish line. Only then will we see what is on the other side. It's just a journey to get where God needs you. Lord, I pray for endurance for each and every one of us. Wherever we are at in our battle. Give us peace, joy, and comfort in knowing that you guide our each and every step.
God Bless,
Debbie

Just finding your inner beauty does not make everything well; it is just a part of the grand overhaul, part of the damage reversal. I had just spent so much of my time fighting the cancer that my self-image had to be put on hold. Focusing on my physical appearance would have been like trying to redecorate my home while it was on fire. I felt like Scarlett O'Hara in *Gone with the Wind* saying, "I can't think about this right now, I'll think about this tomorrow."

You must have a strategy for what is right in front of you. At that moment, for me, chemotherapy was what had most of my attention, and that was how it had to be. Cancer was a breeze: just cut it out. It was the precautionary stuff that was killing me. Ironically, each step closer to death meant that I was that much closer to life. Ten months ago, I'd told the doctor to go as aggressively as possible with my treatments because I did not want to come back to this place ever again. I'm glad I made that decision early on, before I started the treatments, because once you're in it, it starts to feel like a bad idea. My body was physically torn, worn, and battered, and all my mom could do was to try and make me as comfortable as possible.

Hey Guys,

The side effects are less severe this time around because they cut my dose by 25%. I have sores on my hands and in my mouth but praise God not on my feet. My blood count is gone again and my blood pressure is 98/51. However, all this is not out of the norm. I'm not experiencing more than the average person. The word I keep receiving is stand and then stand again and when you're done, stand some more. My father recently asked me if I was starting to get bitter. Absolutely not. That has never entered my mind. I do experience sadness and weariness but who says that's a bad place? That is exactly where God steps in. I am however left without words at this point. I pray in the spirit because I'm tired and my spirit is better equipped at this point to stand. Once I let my spirit go for it, I was taken back by the power and strength that poured out. It was exhilarating. Dedicate 15 minutes to praying in the spirit every day. I know some of you already do but for those of you who don't, go for it. I have often heard of the Holy Spirit as the comforter, and after years of being a Christian, I now know. It amazes me on how much we hear but never experience.

God Bless,
Debbie.

In one of my puny attempts at not accepting where I was physically, I tried to go out and do some motherly type errands, even though I had a feeling that this was going to end badly, which, by the way, it did. I started off at 7:00 a.m. and everything felt fine but by 2:00 in the afternoon, I was at home, crying in pain, an all-over kind of pain, a nothing-you-could-do type of pain, it was a reeling type of pain I had never felt before. Ten hours later, at 2:00 in the morning, I was driving myself to the emergency room in tears because I was too embarrassed to call anyone to drive me because I had pushed myself too hard when I knew better. I felt so stupid because once again I'd tried to call the shots and determine what I could and could not do. Control is one of those little attributes that I was still struggling with and trying to get a handle on. It took five long days of hospitalization to bounce back.

Interestingly, this was the week that Hurricane Katrina hit the Louisiana Gulf Coast, which in turn, really hindered my ability to feel sorry for myself. The hurricane coverage was the only thing on television, and no matter how hard I tried to put a spin on my situation, all I could feel was how blessed I was to be in that hospital, receiving the care that I needed. Isolation can play tricks on your mind, and I was definitely born to favor human contact. Yet the only contact that I would receive would be when a nurse would come in once about every four to five hours, completely masked and in a sterile gown, to check my vitals. Three times a day, an aide would leave a tray of food by the door, and once a day, a masked person would empty the trash. I missed everyone.

By the fourth day, I was missing my children badly but, with a no-visitor order, seeing them was not going to happen. I was having a *Terms of Endearment* moment, thinking about my kids coming in to visit; I was picturing the scene in the movie when her boys came in to say goodbye just before she died. Having a personality that is a bit on the dramatic side, my imagination was having a field day. It did not help that I was looking more and more like that woman in the movie, complete with that ashy, death-colored skin. In fact, I looked even worse because remember, I had no hair, eyelashes, or eyebrows.

Just as I was about to go for it emotionally with an Academy Award-winning moment, my cousin, who happens to be a pastor, called, and just in the knick of time, he was able to bring me back to the reality of my situation, which was actually a pretty great place to be because I was almost done. I was at the tail end of my own personal hurricane. It would have been a complete shame to lose it right at the last minute. I could not allow the loneliness to move me in the wrong direction. Loneliness is a whopper of an emotion to try and get through.

27

Once the Stone Hits the Water, You Can't Stop the Ripples

It had been over two and a half years since I had been involved with a man in any way, shape, or form. I had not even received a phone call or a spark of interest from anyone of the male persuasion. It's definitely not a good feeling when you come to the realization that your whole life has been spent looking to a man for validation as a woman, or as anything for that matter. However, I had predetermined to have no involvement with men until my divorce was final. Integrity takes a lot of work, and as long as I was still married, I was determined to conduct myself as such. But, my goodness, I wasn't even given the opportunity to say, "Oh no, I'm so sorry, I just can't accept your invitation for a candle-lit dinner and a romantic movie because I'm just not ready yet." Somehow, I'd had it in my mind that being married meant wholeness. But in my particular case, it was just a mirage, not a marriage.

As a God-given leader, I should have been extremely careful, because leaders can easily get carried away with their gifting and try to lead their own lives, and that is God's job, not ours. A leader is to lead others as a guide or as a director. We can lose control over being in control. I had always taken charge over my own life, which closed out the ability for God to move. Because I was a leader, I thought I could fix the chaos in my life when, in reality, I was the one who had caused it by taking control in the first place.

Being the only girl of three children, I was very pampered. O.K., spoiled. If I wanted it, my parents did their best to bless me with it; in other words, I almost always got what I wanted. Well, as an adult, it became a problem. Some things are just not meant to be yours. The ripple effect that you cause by taking things that do not belong to you is massive and endless. The damage that I had caused from destroying my first marriage was still being suffered by my seventeen-year-old son, in ways that I could never have imagined.

My first husband's family had issues with me even before the bad breakup. Fairly early on in the marriage I was told that Paul had married beneath him so you can only imagine what a bad taste I left in their mouths after the messy and scandalous divorce. A perfect example of the ripple effect happened once, while my son was at a family gathering with his father's side of the family, and one of his cousins told him that I was getting everything I deserved. My son was devastated and hurt, and quickly came to my defense. However, because of my actions, my son was still being affected thirteen years later. That was seed that I had sown. Those are people whom I still negatively impact to this very day. I strive to live with integrity and to never again be moved by loneliness or desperation. My desperation to be loved has cost me enough of life's happiness as it is. I walk away from my past by changing my future. The control I proudly take responsibility for is handing my life over to God. So, on we go to chemo treatment number nine.

Here We Go!
Hey Guys,
Be blessed today. I go for chemo today. All is good. Let me rephrase that, all is awesome, I am truly blessed. God is so in my face. I can't imagine life any other way. To all of you, I am so proud and blessed to call you friend, no, to call you family.
God Bless,
Debbie

Just when I thought that I had a handle on things, once again, I was proven wrong. You'd think that I would get tired of making things worse and that I would stop trying to figure out how to adjust to the effects of chemo. This new medicine was just too rough to recover from; when I would start to see the light of day, BAM, it was time to go back for another treatment.

I knew deep down in my bones that more hospital time was coming. I felt like I was in a walking coma. Every once in a while, I would come across something that would warm my heart, like the time when I went into my younger daughter's bedroom to put some clothes away and sitting on her bed, propped up on her pillow, was one of her Barbie dolls. My older daughter had cut off all of her hair; the Barbie was completely bald. When I asked why she had done it, she said, "Because I wanted her to be as beautiful as you." My goodness, what do you say to that? You would be surprised at how something that honest and true will get you through another day. At this point, I was grabbing on to anything and everything for whatever glimmer of hope or joy I could find. Sickness has a funny way of helping you find that desperation for God.

Webster's New World Dictionary defines the word "desperate" as having a very great desire or need, extreme, drastic, without hope.

There was nothing I could do but sit back and pray my way through the battle with this disease. This cup wasn't going anywhere.

O.K. Nine down and down Is What I Did, Flat on My Face

Hey Everyone!
I miss you all so much. I feel like the kid that got benched and they won't let me back in the game. So, as some of you know this last chemo was a whopper. After being down for six days I landed myself a four-day stay in the hospital. I was minus white blood cells and I managed to catch something which I was unable to fight on my own. Who said the devil would go down quietly? I say let him make all the noise he wants, he is still going down. O.K. Yes, by the third day I was crying a river again but my pastor says that this is not a sign of defeat. I like to think of it as, watering all of the seeds that I've planted as well as watering all of the seed that many of you have planted in us. Besides, I know that I am one of God's favorites. How do I know that? Among all the truly amazing things God has done and continues to do for us on a daily basis, this morning, while sitting on my hospital bed, I received a phone call from my church. I do not mean before church or after church, I mean during church, from the pulpit, the

pastor pulled out his cell phone and called me in the middle of service so
that the whole church could say hello, and they prayed for me all together.
Yes, my Father spoils me. One hour later, I was released from the hospital.
We're blessed in the city
We're blessed in the fields
We're blessed when we come and when we go.
Is God completely awesome or what?
So the bottom line is ONLY ONE MORE TREATMENT!
I love you,
Debbie

Believe it or not, I was still trying to get Michael to go and sign the divorce papers so that I could officially close that chapter in my life. I just found it hard to swallow that I would finish cancer before getting my release from this guy. Something always seemed to come up, and he wouldn't make it. He had made a few attempts but there were always mistakes that nullified the paperwork. I looked at all of the obstacles as a tactic of the enemy. I don't believe that the divorce was being held up on purpose. I do believe that Michael wanted this behind him just as much as I did; his new life was well under way. It was the devil's way of trying to get me to bite and start fighting.

Up to this point, we had still managed to not go off on each other. I was dodging all kinds of hooks that were trying to gouge at me and drag me into battle, but this tactic was not going to work on me anymore. I had formed a million opinions on how my husband, his girlfriend, and my girls were interacting with one another, opinions that I forced myself to sit on. I would hear something that was said or done while the girls were on their visit with their father, and I wanted to jump right on the phone and give him a piece of my mind. I would become so enraged that I'd lose all rationale to the point of ridiculousness that would then snap me back to reality, allowing me to realize that this was one of those hooks that I had referred to, and had I made that call, I would have played right into the hands of the enemy.

It was not Michael or his girlfriend trying to hook me, it was the devil; he had been trying to get me to call them and engage in battle for over two years, but I would not call them; I would pray. It was not my place to control his relationship with his girls; as long as they were not being mentally or physically abused anymore, I had to let it go. He loved his girls, and it was not my place to try to dictate their life with their dad. I knew that if I'd opened that door that the door would then swing both ways, and I was not going to invite him to voice his opinions or speak anything into my life in any way, shape, or form. I was fighting chemo with everything I had in me; I could not seem to muster up the oomph that was needed to badger him about why he would not make the divorce a priority. But finally, the constant phone calls and constant pressure from my attorney paid off, because he made an appointment and actually went to see her. The Lord had told me that once the cancer and the divorce had run their course, this book would be finished. I finally started to feel that they were both nearing completion. I was at a complete loss for words regarding the direction in which the book had taken. I'd set out to journal my divorce, and it ended up being so much more. But, just like a good movie, with all the twists and turns, I would not, could not understand all of it until the end.

28

Today I Declare Victory
Because I Didn't Quit

Last But Not Least

Hey Guys,
Today will mark the change from search and rescue to search and recovery. Any last bit of cancer that may exist in my body will die today. Today I look death in the face, smile, and walk away. I feel like an Olympian in first place with my arms straight up to the sky and I can see the ribbon about to hit my chest. I know on this day my Father is well pleased. Death was never an option, I was told by three prophets that life would be my prize. First by Lydia Suesoff then by E. Vann Walker and then by Ed Traut. My body hasn't fully recovered from the last chemo so I'm not sure what to expect on this last treatment; however, we are taking extra precautions this time around. I am looking forward to recovery. God told me that I would get back everything that I'd lost. This time around I will use my life to first further the kingdom. I will also purpose never to lose sight of God and His continuous blessings in my life. I first live to please God, second for His will in my life, and third for the lives of my children. I have not lived through a season of divorce and cancer. I have lived through a season of love. God has lavished me through my family, friends, and my church. God has never left my side for a moment. I have fallen in love with God and also have learned and lived His love for me. It has definitely cost me but I must say it has been the best investment of my life. I have not found God through the

storm, I found Him in spite of it. He truly is my rock.
God Bless You and Your Family,
Debbie

So as you may have guessed, I ended up back in the hospital, blah, blah, blah. So what?! I was done. I got as sick as ever but I never lost faith. Do you have any idea how completely awesome it feels to say that?! I never lost faith. Say it with me, "I NEVER LOST FAITH!" Yes, I had a hard time doing everything; climbing a flight of stairs, I was hurting in places that I didn't even know could hurt, but I never lost faith. For the second time within three years, in the midst of a great storm, I stood. Yes, I looked like complete and total hell but I was walking away from death. Actually, it was more like crawling away, but "away" is the operative word.

While I was still in the hospital, I received word that all of my divorce papers were at last completed and were awaiting my final signature before filing. I had waited almost three years to hear those words but I was too sick to do anything about it. It would take me another four weeks before I was strong enough to go to meet with my attorney and sign on the dotted line. I was so completely amazed at how thoroughly trashed my body felt.

Now began the waiting game; I had to wait for my divorce to be final. I had to wait for my body to rejuvenate. I had to wait for everything to grow back and I had to wait for this book to be finished. I had to wait for reconstructive surgery, even to just put make-up on. Come on ladies, you know that some of you would have been presumed dead or missing in action if you were unable to put on make-up for one whole year. The point is, I had to wait for everything.

I remember that one of my best friends blessed me with $40 to go out and buy my favorite Lancôme compact. I had started using nothing but Lancôme at the age of nineteen, but for the last ten years I could no longer afford it. I had held on to that $40 for four weeks because I was not sure if my skin would react negatively or not. I'd kept the money in my car visor and would pull it out every so often but would slip it back until I felt the time was right. My skin tone had changed so much that I knew I would literally have to try the make-up on my face to find my new color.

Finally I felt it was time. I went to Robinson's May so excited, I felt giddy. I was so sure that the timing was right, I was actually singing songs in my head and walking with a bounce. I told the representative all about what I had been through and told her how excited I was to see if my skin would react negatively or not. She held up different shades to my skin, trying to match my face. I was still bald, so it had to match my head as well. When you go bald from chemo and are restricted from the sun, your scalp and face do not get a chance to meld together. When she started to apply the make-up, it started to show all the flaky dead skin; I had developed deep crevasses, but hey, no problem, I will just have to exfoliate more often.

The representative was starting to look nervous. She kept trying to smooth out the rough spots but it was not working. When I looked in the mirror, it looked like I had a mask on because there was no hairline to work the color into. Then, as I sat there, looking in the mirror, trying to figure out how to make it meld, my skin started to react very badly. The stress of it all then threw me into a hot flash of massive proportions, which in turn brought on ridiculous sweats. As I stared in the mirror, realizing that it was not going to work, my face was turning a bright shade of red and was literally hot to the touch. The tears started flowing slowly down my face, into the crevasses, and making dramatic lines in the make-up. The representative did not know what to say, and I could tell that she wanted to cry with me. My sorrow was deep. I simply touched her hand and said, "It's O.K. Really, it's going to be O.K.…. It's just not time yet." I took the tissue from her hand and started to wipe off the make-up. I got up from the chair and walked out with my head held purposely up high, but when I got into my car I just sat there and cried into my hands for a couple of minutes. After I'd gotten it all out, I quietly slipped the money back into the visor and decided to put it out of my mind. I don't know if a man can relate to this experience. For about thirty minutes, I'd actually felt as if I were going to be able to somewhat fix my face but it just wasn't time.

Are We Finished Yet?
Jesus, Jesus, Jesus, Jesus, Jesus, Jesus, Jesus, Jesus, Oh, sorry, I got carried away. But as you all know, there is power in the name of Jesus. This last week there were times that the name Jesus was all that would come out

of my mouth. And as I have come to know, that is all I needed to get me through. I no longer can see the finish line unless I look back over my shoulder. It is just that my feet got tangled up in the finish line ribbon. I am back up on two feet but will use wisdom in my recovery. There is no doubt that this body has had it. Now just sit back and watch what God can do. My God makeover is done on the inside. Now it's time for the outside. I feel like introducing myself to you all over again because the person I am today is completely new. Maybe not new, just recently discovered.
I love you, and God Bless,
Debbie

29

Now I Had to Assess the Damage

Now that I had chemo behind me, I had to face the aftermath, and I had to tend to it. My first priorities in what I had to contend with were my children, because for the past year they had basically been raising themselves. I was able to remember things that had happened, which at the time I had been unable to either address or comprehend, good as well as bad. I remember once while driving, it hit me that in the midst of chemotherapy, I'd tried to direct a play. God kept trying to throw up road blocks but in my tunnel vision, I could only keep forging ahead. I had people dropping out or not showing up for rehearsal, and the people who were showing up were getting bothered by those who would not learn lines, and I even had a leading cast member incarcerated for two months.

I finally conceded that maybe God was trying to tell me something, so I reluctantly surrendered and I told God, "O.K. I get it." Now that I was done with chemo, I had a chance to reflect; I sat in the car asking myself if that really happened. I called our church administrator and asked him, "Did I really try and direct a play during chemo?" I thought maybe I was getting my years messed up but, no, that was not the case. I actually tried to do it. I rehearsed for two months before I would finally surrender.

Another thing that I realized was that my son had gone to New York over Easter vacation with his drama class. We were walking out of the movies when it hit me; I then turned and hit him on the shoulder and said, "You went to New York when I was in the middle of chemo? Are you kidding me?" It was funny because even in my darkest state, I could not stop being a mother; I could only think of him not missing out on an incredible opportunity.

Now, I was listening to my kids fighting over everything. My mom had basically lived with us since the discovery of the cancer, and she began fighting right along with them; she even sounded like them. They were all barking out orders at each other, and no one was listening to anyone; just the volume alone was irritating. I knew that this was a direct result of my mental absence for the last ten months, and it was going to take some serious work to regain control of it all. They had to know that I was back, and I had to rescue my mom. She was no longer equipped to be a mother of young children and was very content in being the grandma who got to go home and leave the madness behind. I started sending her home so that she could start to regain her life. We all needed to regain a sense of normalcy.

It was hard taking the control back from my kids but once I did, I think even they were relieved. The thing that helped the most was one day, my big brother called and said that he had a dining room table that he needed to get rid of and asked if I wanted it. My table was in really bad shape, with a big black iron mark on it, so I gratefully jumped at the offer. It was big, beautiful, and elegant but we had no chairs to match, so we got whatever chairs we had and put them around our new table. We even used outdoor plastic chairs to fill in the empty places. Normally at dinner, everyone ate wherever they wanted with a T.V. tray in front of whatever T.V. they could find. This meant that everyone was spread out all over the house. Well, now, since we had this great, big table, I wanted to try something new. We all ate together. Imagine that: at the same time, without a T.V., and we would actually attempt to talk.

The first three nights were disastrous. Our usual cast of characters included my three kids, my mom, my son's father, and me. There was fighting, crying, and usually someone wanting to leave the table because no one was listening to them. I remember once someone shouting, "We need a lawyer!" and I remember thinking, I don't know if all of this was going to be worth the extreme effort. My son's father and my mom would say, "I'm out of here."

But on the fourth night, something miraculously changed, and the fourth night was great. It took a minute, but only because we had not learned, as a family, to sit together and respect one another, to really listen and care about what the others had to say. I know it sounds basic and simplistic yet it was something that had been overlooked in our family. We'd never before done it, ever, not through the span of two marriages, which consisted of twenty-five years in total. In fact, I had never in my life sat at a table with my family unless it was a holiday or special occasion.

By the fifth night, everyone met at the table with excitement and eager anticipation. We had already given up fast food due to a lack of money, and I was cooking homemade food. Aside from the obvious heath benefits, the added perk was that everyone preferred my cooking anyway. We were bonding a little more with each and every meal, and it was great. It gave us the opportunity to give to each other without any outside distractions; I really enjoyed that time with my family. Sometimes in the past, things would get so hectic throughout the day that we would not even get a chance to look each other in the eyes, but not any more. I would like to thank my brother David for the table. It meant more than you'll ever know.

30

It Was Time to Speak
It from My Mouth

E-Mail Alert

I just came back from the doctor's office.
IT IS OFFICIAL!
THIS HOUSE IS CLEAN!!!!
I AM CANCER FREE!
WOW! NOW LET'S GET
ABOUT GOD'S BUSINESS!
I'd waited so long to hear those words.

Twice in the last couple of months, I had been asked if I wanted to give a praise report at church. I was so full of gratitude but I did not want to speak until I could say that the cancer was gone. Well, that day finally came, and it was time for me to speak with my mouth. Everyone had watched me for ten months, moving in faith, and now it was time to hear it in words. I was welcomed with such an embrace of cheers and clapping that I felt as if we were all celebrating a grand victory as one. I knew that these would be my first steps into my new destiny.

I spoke for fifteen minutes, and although I would get overwhelmed at times, the Lord helped me to get out what I needed to. I shared my heart with my family and my church. The main thing that I wanted to say after "thank you" was that, contrary to my situation and what I physically looked like, I was quite possibly in the best place I had ever been. We, my kids and I, were in the best place **WE** had ever been in. I shared with the congregation about living the seasons of love and how not to give your temporary situation power over how you choose to live life, how walking with God means walking in love, and that man cannot dictate your future unless you give him your power. Situations cannot defeat you unless you give up. My children and I stood up in front of our church, united, joyful, and soaring. The devil had given us his best shot, and we were still standing, not only standing but standing stronger than ever, each one of us flourishing in our own right. We literally shined. My girls sang the song *Seasons of Love* from the Broadway musical *Rent*: "In daylights, in sunsets, in midnights, in cups of coffee."

I had learned to find love using all my five senses: sight, sound, taste, touch, and smell. I could see the work of God's hand in the brilliance of a sunset, I could hear God's love in the laughter of my children, I could taste it in the richness of a chocolate kiss, I could feel it in the warmth of the sun on my face, and I could smell it in a flower.

I had learned to find God in everything, and I learned to draw strength from anything that came my way, in songs from Cher, Nellie Furtado, Nora Jones, and a lot from Christina Aguilera. Christina and I spent the most time together because her songs covered the full spectrum of my four-year struggle, from *Fighter* to *Beautiful* to *Soar* which she wrote. I felt like I knew that whoever had written those songs had once been where I had been. Even Kelly Clarkson was empowering with *Since You've Been Gone*. Of course, I always had praise and worship music on hand as well. It was a way for me to get the word in my spirit while driving.

The books I delved into were exceptional as well. I read *The Purpose Driven Life* by Rick Warren, *The Prayer of Jabez* by Dr. Bruce H. Wilkinson, *Praying God's Will for Your Life* by Stormie Omartian, *The Traveler's Gift* by Andy Andrews, *Woman Thou Art Loosed* by T.D. Jakes, *The Ultimate Survivor* by Frieda White, *God's Favorite House* by Tommy Tenney, *Battlefield of the Mind* by Joyce Meyer, and *Boundaries* by Dr. Henry Cloud and Dr. John Townsend. These books and songs helped me in regaining my power. I am naming these titles specifically because if you are finding yourself in a battle, you may need some suggestions on where to start towards your fighting back, because you must be proactive and do your part.

I found God in friends, in work, in strangers, and even in movies; the movie *Diary of a Mad Black Woman* was a good one. I suggest sitting back for a moment and looking around; there are signs of God's love for you everywhere you look; it is right in front of your face. Seek God and you will find God. It is as simple as that.

I would like to make it clear that even when fighting the good fight, there will definitely be black times, those dark moments when you cry all alone. The trick is in fighting through those times instead of getting stuck there. I was back to the business of reconstructing my life while God brought back all that I had lost. Still, my regrets had a tendency to wreak havoc on my mental state, almost to a paralyzing place. I was so sorry that I had not developed deeper friendships, because for the past three years, I'd only confided in three people, and even that was usually just by phone. The first year and a half, I was dealing with heartbreak as well as a broken spirit, and I did not want to see anyone. Then the second year and a half, I was dealing with cancer and chemo, and I could not see anyone. The reality was that I had pushed everyone away for whatever reason a long time ago. Now that I could really use some close, personal friends, I had nothing to draw from.

The few that I did have were understandably worn out. The book I read entitled *Boundaries* explained about having a circle or an array of friends, not just a couple or three but many, like a bouquet of friends. People have full lives and unintentionally are not always available. I am definitely not talking about the stereotypical high school friendships, which consume each others' lives, but occasional, trustworthy, healthy friendships. Here I was, ready to enjoy life with people, and there was no one there, at least that is how I perceived it.

When my kids would leave for their weekend visits with their father, I would purposely not call people to see if my phone would ring, and guess what? It wouldn't. I did it for three consecutive weeks, and every time, I had the same results. I had abandoned my friends years ago when I got married to Michael, and then he turned around and abandoned me and our marriage. I could not seem to shake that "reap what you sow" business. It would've been so easy to blame people and to be hurt but that kind of thinking is simply not rational, because unless you open yourself up to one another, you will always find yourself alone. I wasn't longing for a man; I was longing for people, good and loving people, but I had not sown the seeds of friendship that are required in order to receive those blessings. The problem was that I was ready to get back into life, and I had not yet shared that with anyone.

My older brother invited me to his house for his annual work Christmas party. Every year, he invites his friends from work to his home. Going to my brother's house during the Christmas season is an experience in itself; everything is elegant and beautiful, but just add the warmth and love of friends, and it becomes awesome. At the party, I sat back and watched the procession as people came in, one right after another. The women were dressed seasonally and festive, and the men looked very handsome and debonair; everyone was so glad just to be there, and each person brought a dish to add to the beautiful buffet.

As I watched my brother move from person to person, making sure that everyone had what they needed, I thought to myself, "He's got it; he learned something that I had missed. He is relational; my brother knows how to be a part of people because he experiences life past his own little world." God has instructed us to love one another, and we are to minister to one another through those relationships. It most certainly does not stop with your spouse and children. I was a woman who thought that that was all she needed, but I'd had it all wrong. God never said to love one person and then stop. He said to love thy neighbor as thy self, so why is it then that people don't enjoy each other more often?

Why are people so critical and hurtful as opposed to nurturing and loving? My brother has a minimum of three Christmas parties a year just to fit in all of the people in his life. There is one for co-workers, one for close friends, and one for our family, which grows bigger every year. I overheard people at my brother's party talking about how awesome it was just to make it onto his guest list.

I want to be relational. I want physical, tangible people in my life. I will not try to buy anyone else's love ever again. I am a great person to be a part of, and that should be enough for anyone, and if it is not, then I will move on. I will never again change who I am in order to be loved. I know what it is to be mistreated and abused; now I want to know what it is to be loved and appreciated. I want relationships with people who will help raise my standards to help me become the kind of person that I aspire to be. I want to learn the things that people have to teach me and I also want to impart my gifts with encouragement and joy into the lives of others.

31

A New Understanding
of Life

When I came out of my chemo coma, as I like to call it, I found my finances disastrous; had it not been for my father and my mother, I would have lost everything: my car, my home, as well as my medical insurance. My parents had been carrying me physically, emotionally, and financially for quite some time, and it was time for me to take responsibility for myself as well as my children. Child support for my girls was sporadic and minuscule; meanwhile, the bills I had acquired were monstrous. I was determined to do the right thing and pay my bills. I wanted to become a responsible adult who my parents and my children would be proud of.

I went back to work full time at our family business, and this time I actually worked. When you work for your family, you have greater leeway to do as you please. I did not want to take advantage of my family like that anymore. I became accountable to my mother as well as my brother Dennis, and them to me. I never just took off to do my own thing, which is what I was used to. I always let them know where I was going, and I always came back. I cut down on personal phone calls during work hours, and I did not talk to my friends while they were working. I paid my bills and I bought my own food, which meant that there wasn't money for anything else. We used to go out to dinner four or five times a week. Now maybe we went once a week if we were good. At restaurants, we ordered water instead of soft drinks to keep the bill down, and I would share meals whenever possible. We were cutting every corner just to make ends meet, and now that it was Christmas, this also meant no presents, no tree, no frills, and no extras. Manicures, pedicures, perfumes, Lancôme, or anything that was not a necessity was just added to the long list of wishes. I knew that this lesson was all part of the bigger picture of a new and more meaningful way of life. I had never, ever not given gifts, and what made this particularly hard was that I knew people were buying gifts for us. I was determined for us to get the meaning of this Christmas right.

I explained it to my kids in the best way that I could, and they didn't care about all the frills and the stuff. They took it much easier than I did. The week before Christmas, I was literally shaking with the desire to go out and buy presents in any way that I could, yet I knew that if I were to do that, I would lose the point of what God truly wanted us to experience this holiday season. I only felt a release in my spirit to purchase just one present, and that was to be for my older brother David. I had learned so much from watching him at his party, and I wanted him to know how much I appreciated him in my life. I cried so many times about not being able to give gifts to all of the people who I loved, until I finally accepted the fact and realized that it was me who had the meaning of Christmas all twisted. It wasn't so much my kids who had to get it about Christmas being about the birth of Christ; it was me.

One night, on our way to dinner with my family, my younger daughter asked if she could borrow my flashlight because she wanted to write down her thoughts in the car and it was dark. I felt that it was odd for her to put it that way, so adult-like, but I smiled and complied with her request. What she wrote was a letter about Christmas, and she read it to us at dinner.

It read:

> To me the main reason about celebrating Christmas is about Jesus being born. It is not about presents or lights. So, if you think celebrating Christmas is about lights, Christmas trees, and presents, you're wrong. Do you know if Jesus wasn't born we wouldn't be so happy? So, get happy and celebrate Christmas because Jesus is born. Author: Tiffany

She understood; we didn't have a tree, presents, lights, or any physical sign of a typical Christmas at our home, and at nine years old, she got what it took me over forty years to get. All three of my children did. The best present I could give them was me being here; I'd fought and worked hard for my life, and this was what I had to give to them. There are many women who have died from breast cancer, and I was not one of them. My parents were spared the loss of their daughter, my brothers, the loss of their only sister, my kids, the loss of their mom, and my friends were spared the loss of a friend. This Christmas could have ended disastrously, but then God stepped in.

This was the most beautiful and meaningful Christmas of our lives. I think the greatest aspect of this particular Christmas was that it fell on Sunday. On Sunday morning, we were in church, praising, worshiping, and celebrating the birth of Christ. This is what I gave my children this particular year: The true meaning of Christmas, and it will be up to them to keep it. As for me, I will never forget the Christ in Christmas for as long as I live.

As I sit back and look at myself on a deeper level, I find that there are many things that I walked away from that I regret and miss. When I married for the second time, I walked away from everything and everyone who had anything to do with who I had been. I then allowed my new husband Michael to mold me into what he felt I should be, from my hair style to the clothes that I wore. He liked curly hair, t-shirts, and sweats, so I got a perm and dressed down. I had become the epitome of a people pleaser, or at least a one-person pleaser. I did whatever it took to insure his love for me.

I remember early on in our involvement, I was going through a lot of pictures of old friends, most of which were guys, and because they made him feel uncomfortable, I chose to throw them away. I got rid of all my memorabilia from concerts and my playbills from Broadway show that I had seen because if he didn't find them important, then neither should I. My past behavior is difficult and embarrassing to admit to. I so wanted to be a part of something that had no place for me; that something was Michael's heart.

I remember once, he was having a tattoo marathon at our house. The artist was tattooing all of the guys for free. After all the guys were done getting their "ink" and left for the music studio, I tattooed my husband's name over my heart. If you were to have met me in person, you wouldn't have thought that I would be the type to get a tattoo. I was far too un-hip, and honestly, it was something that had never even entered my mind. It was one of the most out-of-character things I had ever done. I just figured that no one would ever see it. I also think it was another way for me to try and make myself more permanent in his life and he in mine.

I admit this only because, if any of you find yourselves in a similar place, I need you to know that you are not alone; it can happen to the best of us. Surrendering my identity was never about how awesome I thought he was, because no human's presence should ever draw anyone into abandoning who you are. Sacrificing yourself is more about how completely unworthy you see yourself, about how ugly you feel on the inside. It is about not liking yourself and being willing to do whatever it takes to be loved. God did not give us the capacity to love one another with the idea that we should end up paying for it.

I remember about a month after Michael left me, I was standing up at the altar in church, professing to God that He was Lord over my life, and then I remembered the tattoo. I thought, "Here I stand saying that my life belongs to God and yet I have tattooed a man's name over my heart." I can only imagine what you must be thinking: "How astronomically stupid." I just wanted to kick myself. And ironically, it was not on the breast that I lost to cancer. No, that would have been too easy. Talk about paying for your mistakes, I would have to endure three years of laser treatments to remove his name. I just couldn't seem to catch a break. I would go in once every two months to have a technician use a machine that shot out a red laser beam that would attempt to blast the tattoo out of my skin. The first treatment that I received was without any anesthesia to numb the pain, and I had to wear goggles to protect my eyes from the beam. I could smell the burning flesh; it instantaneously swelled and afterward looked like an open pomegranate with a lot of tiny blisters.

My cousin had taken me to the appointment, and I remember going to a restaurant afterwards and sitting there in shock. I just sat there staring at him. This was much bigger than just removing a tattoo. Then I started crying because it felt like it was one more stronghold that I was able to have broken over my life. I was one step closer to regaining Deborah. So, I kept up with the treatments until the tattoo was gone. There were times it would bleed right through the bandage, bra, and shirt. And who would have thought that it would take three years? One never truly knows the price until it comes time to pay.

32

All That Being Said,
It Is Still on You!

You have heard that hindsight is 20/20, and as I sit here and go over it all, my life, I can no longer say that this is all because of what someone said or did to me. I thought I had come up with the answer as to why my life had spiraled out of control and into such devastation. I had this self-revelation that all of the destruction began on the day that my first husband Paul, sat me down and told me, completely out of the blue, after five years of marriage, that he didn't think that he could be married to me for life. Yes, it sounds bad, and I am sure that there were all kinds of extenuating circumstances, but the truth of the matter is, that was just not a good enough reason to abandon who I was and turn my back on everything that I stood for. There will never be a reason, or should I say any excuse, good enough for diving head first into sin because when you stand before God, the "he said, she said" notion is just not going to fly.

The truth was that the words of my first husband were not what threw me into a tailspin; it was that I had never learned to become a whole person or an individual. I had always looked for my validation in a man, and when Paul pulled the rug out from under me and that relationship was no longer stable, I fell apart, as I had my whole life. I did, however, find his hurtful words useful years later when I used them as an excuse to follow temptation and have an affair, and I even had the audacity to say that he was the one who drove me to do it. When I was able to rationalize that he had driven me into the arms of someone else, it somehow took the pressure and responsibility off of me. In my mind, it became his fault because he was not watching over his nest. There is no way that one statement should have ruined an eleven-year marriage unless I was looking for an excuse to end it. Besides, we had made it through another six years of marriage, which included the birth of our son, after his damaging words. So, when temptation came knocking, six years is how far back I had to reach in order to find a big enough excuse to blame someone else for what I was about to do. I felt that his cruel words gave me free license to now say, because he hurt me so badly then, that I now have the right to reach out and take a bite of that apple. I was looking for excuses coming and going.

It is funny how people have a tendency to think of Adam and Eve as weak. People like to think that they would have never bitten that apple, but the apple simply represents sin. Let he who is without sin cast the first stone. You know, some of us would be better off putting a lid on it and just go and make a few apple pies with all of the apples we have bitten; in my case, throw in some apple preserves as well. When my life was spiraling out of control, God kept throwing out safety nets to try and save me, but I kept dodging them because I wanted what I wanted, period. It was as if I was falling down a huge hole and all the way down, there were all kinds of nets from God trying to help me, but because I was so twisted, I saw them as the snares of the enemy, trying to trap me and keep me from what I wanted, never realizing that had I just grabbed onto one of them, God would have been able to step in on my behalf. I was unable to distinguish between God and the serpent. I had inadvertently reached for the devil instead of God. I had completely mixed them up.

Once I embraced temptation, the devil was able to deceive me. He is the father of all lies; never forget that that is his little job title. To think that you are above being deceived by the devil will be your first mistake. I will never again say, "He made me do it," or "She made me go," or "They confused me," or "He just got me so mad that I had to react." I will not act out of emotion, which is a huge accomplishment in itself because I am an emotional being. I will not be pulled into things that bring harm or destruction into my life or the lives of those around me. I will not be moved by insecurity, and I will not let being alone (without a man) move me. I have made it to a place of completion within myself, as a woman, through God.

You can always look for and find excuses to do whatever it is that you want. My point is that if it is of God, you do not need an excuse. Review your past as a way to learn from it, not relive it. Find where you made mistakes and why you made those bad decisions, do your best not to justify them, because that will only hold you up longer. I had convinced myself, for over sixteen years, that I had been driven by someone else to do what I did. I blamed my first husband for my circumstance; therefore, I was unable to learn from my true mistake, which was that I had simply said "yes" to sin. Until I took ownership of my own sin, I was unable to give it to God because you cannot give what does not belong to you.

That is what it means to work out your own salvation. Stop trying to put your stuff on someone else. It only prolongs your pain.

I will not use my past abuses, hurts, or disappointments as a crutch or an excuse for bad decisions. As an adult, I can see that as a child I was wronged, and that because of those hurts and abuses, I am the way I am, but now as an adult I have the power to change what I now see clearly as dysfunctional. I need to learn from my past and stop reliving it over and over. When I do decide on something, it will be because it was a well-thought-out and confident decision that I made for myself with the help of my heavenly Father.

33

Back to Life

Believe it or not, it had been three years since Michael had walked out on us, and I was still waiting for my divorce to become final. Everything had been filed, and all I could do was wait. I thought that maybe I would receive my papers for Thanksgiving, but no such luck. Then I thought what an incredible gift it would be if I were to receive my papers for Christmas. So two days before Christmas, my cell phone began to ring; my caller I.D. read "Attorney." I got chills and filled with excitement, but to no avail. It was my attorney, but she was only calling to wish me a Merry Christmas. When I answered, I didn't even say hello, I answered, "Is it done?" When she said no, I knew that she had detected the sadness and disappointment in my deep, heavy sigh. I told her that it was nothing personal but that I did not want her to call me again unless she had my final papers in her hand, so that the next time I saw her name on my cell, I would know that it was finished.

At the same time that I filed my divorce papers, I was also put on a waiting list for reconstructive surgery. I was using my own body as opposed to an implant, so it was a much more complicated procedure and would require three different surgeries over a six-month period. The first surgery would be the biggest one, with an eight-hour ordeal. I put the surgery and the divorce completely in God's hands and moved on with life the best that I could. Everything that was required from me in both situations was in. I found that waiting on God can sometimes be as aggravating as watching grass grow. It is better to do what is required of you and then come back later after it has had a chance to grow. You can lose a lot of ground when you just sit, watch, and wait. I've learned that once you have done your part, it's best to work on the next task at hand. For me, it was another theatrical production at my church. It was very important for me to have all three of my children right by my side, working together, so I prayed that the Lord would give me something that would include us all. This time, for the first time ever, it was to be a production with children only. I took a musical that was written for nine adults and split all the parts up to use seventeen children. And yes, most definitely, all three of my children were part of the cast. Once we started rehearsals, the production hit a few bumps in the road, as usual. Nothing too out of the norm, and I had become great at saying, "Let's make it work," so there wasn't anything that was going to derail this play. God was very thorough in helping me pick a complete production team. I knew I still had a lot coming down the road with my ever-elusive divorce and my pending surgeries, so instead of waiting for it all to be over, I simply took the necessary precautions and padded everywhere that I thought might be affected by my absence.

In my six previous productions, I'd never had an assistant director, but this time I had three assistants, two producers, a musical director, a couple of choreographers, light people, sound people, property manager; you name it, I HAD IT. So when things unexpected did come up, we would all simply readjust. Satan had nothing on us, we all had learned to bob and weave. We were three months into rehearsals, and I kept having irritating situations in my personal life arise, which were really starting to weigh me down. Things just seemed to be going against me. Like when my attorney finally called; as I stared at my ringing cell phone, I kept reading the word "Attorney" over and over; I had an inner jubilant tingle. After four rings, my phone automatically goes to voice mail, so I waited just before the end of the fourth ring to answer it. Beaming from ear to ear, I answered, slowly yet bubbly, "Hello Julianne, how are you?" With her first word, I knew it wasn't good. She said, "Debbie, I'm sorry. It's not what you want to hear. The divorce did not go through." My body went limp and I simply dropped in my chair at work. I just kept saying no way. No way, I mean, NO WAY. God said that He was in control. What in the world happened now? Julianne told me that the courts had not received Michael's filing fee of $320. Are you kidding me, $320? I just couldn't believe it. It was easier for me to get rid of cancer than it was to get rid of Michael; I mean that literally. I couldn't understand why my husband's girlfriend wasn't giving him more grief about this. Why was there no urgency on their part to right this situation? Why was I the only one hanging onto the edge of my seat for this to be over? I mean, Lord, I don't have to know why on everything you're up to, but please, help me get a clue.

And then it hit me. The reason I was so anxious was because God had told me that with the ending of this marriage would bring my new beginning, which brings me back to leaving it in God's hands. I was so completely frustrated and desperate to get to the other side of this debacle that my human nature spewed out, screaming, go anywhere you can for the $320 to pay his side of the filing fees and just take care of it yourself. Just do it. He will never be held accountable or responsible enough to do it himself, so just handle it, like you always have. Whenever he was in trouble, I got him out. Car impounded, I got it out. Tickets, I paid them. Electricity off, I would come up with the money and get it turned back on. Landlord needed to be called, then I would be the one to make the call; and you know something? I just wasn't going to do that anymore. If it was his responsibility to come up with the money, then by God, that is just what is going to happen. I will not be moved by him or by Satan or by my emotions any longer. It's not my responsibility. This is not my problem to fix. It would have been very easy to move out of position and just do it myself, and as I was going back and forth on my reasoning, God said, rather abruptly, "No, do not be moved. Who told you that this was the end? This is just a status report. You gave this situation over to me. It will be over when I say that it is over. Know that if you take this out of my hands, then it is all back on you." Raise your hand if you know how quickly I dropped that line of questioning. Yes, it took about five seconds. It did, however, leave me with a multitude of emotions to contend with.

Once again, problems seemed to start to pile up and overwhelm me. At one point on this particular Friday, I started to take my own assessment of everything, I mean everything. I even took on stuff that really wasn't mine to carry but since I was piling, I went for it: from not getting my divorce, the delay of my reconstructive surgery, no money, massive bills, my son getting in trouble both in high school as well as possibly being sat down at church, which was a very big deal as far as the play was concerned. I had already lost one of my leads due to bad behavior, and I stood to lose a couple more.

Michael and I were having big problems with parental disagreements, which in turned severed any last ties I had with his side of the family for the time being. My dad was experiencing some very bad things; one friend died from cancer and another received word that his cancer was back.

I could go on and on but I think you get the picture. The bottom line is that I had come to the conclusion that I deserved to get drunk. I know it sounds stupid with all that I had come through but I was trying to soothe and comfort myself. There was no way I was going to turn to a man, which would have been my natural choice fifteen years ago, so I thought, what about alcohol? I thought of something that had worked in the past. I do not have anything against having a drink but when alcohol is used to hide from your situation or to sedate yourself, then yes, most definitely, it is the wrong thing to do. Regardless, I decided to go out and buy a case of beer. Not a six-pack but a case of beer, along with some limes. The kids were gone for the weekend, and I decided that I was going to go for it. I got everything set, and I sat in my living room all night, just looking at the case of beer. I tried so hard to abandon who I was, who I had become, so that I could let loose and go for it. One hour went by, and I had managed to eat a lime, then another hour passed, and then another. I finally fell asleep. In the morning, I thought well, I'll just do it tonight but as you can probably guess, once again, I just couldn't do it. I knew better. I thought it out and saw it as pointless.

Months later, the case of beer was still in my refrigerator. After a while, it became a symbol of my strength because I was able to resist the temptation of alcohol as a vice or excuse. I had learned to deal with my life through prayer, obedience, and having the faith to know that God was in control. Yes, it can be hard and lonely at times, but there are fewer ramifications when you do the right thing. The temporary fix is just not worth the longtime suffering.

So after four months of waiting, I got a call from the hospital that gave me three minutes to decide if I was ready to confirm that in five days I could be ready for the first of three reconstructive surgeries, which was also the eight-hour ordeal. I was completely caught off-guard but had to make an on-the-spot decision right then and there. My exact words to the nurse on the phone were, "Yes … Wait … Umm … NO … Wait a minute … Oh Lord, O.K., yes, let's do it." And just like that, once again, it was time to get everything in order. My backup people at church stepped in with the rehearsals; I paid all the bills, did laundry, and cleaned house. I prepared myself for the up-and-coming pain and the four to six weeks of down time that came with this type of surgery. I knew that more pain was imminent, but I also knew that I was ready for some things to be put back in place. I was ready, but much like labor pains, you never quite understand the intensity of it all until you are there.

I was hospitalized for five days. It took me two days before I could even get up out of bed. I was completely incapacitated. What does that mean? Stitches completely around my breast, across my abdomen, literally from hip to hip, and my body completely swollen like the Pillsbury doughboy. I mean, we are talking hospital gowns, catheterization, and let's not forget the beautiful bedside commode. It would have been utterly impossible to get any more unattractive at this point in my life. So, the cherry on the top of this particular slice of life that I was experiencing, was that every nurse I had was male; not only male, but handsome to boot. Like *Officer and a Gentleman*, Richard Gere-type of looks as well as body. One was named David; I remember when he first came in, my first feeling was horrified as tears came to my eyes. I literally said, verbally, "Are you kidding, a handsome male nurse. Can this get any worse?" He just tried to laugh it off. Then I thought to myself, hey this is like one of those "the glass is half full or half empty" moments. Maybe the Lord said, "She has been through so much already that I'm going to give her the best, including good-looking men to cater to her every need." With that thought, I said, "Come on in, David, join the party." And from that moment on, I felt special. Not special to the nurses but special to God. Do not misunderstand me; the guys were great, and I never felt that they were horrified or disgusted. In fact, over my five-day stay, I developed some great friendships. Don't get me wrong, not the kind of friendship that you keep on going with. Come on now, these guys had seen far too much to be friends, if you know what I mean. However, I do think of them often and pray for them as well as their families.

The doctor wanted me to stay a day or two longer, but I could tell that things were falling apart at home. There was still no contact with my husband's family, so I did not want to call for help. I did not want to reach out to people who were not in my life on a daily basis. I did not want people to come to my aid because of crisis. I figured that you are either in my life or not. I definitely was not going to tell my husband about the surgery. I did not want him to feel sorry for me or give him the satisfaction of being able to come to my aid. Frankly, I would rather have it hard than get help from him. I knew that my children and my mom had had it with each other, and I just had to get home. Somehow, once I was home, I felt their relief. My presence, just sitting on the couch, seemed to calm everyone down.

34

Somehow, I Kept Envisioning the Bride of Frankenstein

By this time, I had lost all sense of modesty, so being that I could hardly move, I had my girls applying the ointments and changing my bandages. They seemed to love having a part in my recovery. However, this makeover was a lot different from all of those makeover shows I had seen on T.V. You know the show that takes a mess of a woman and turns her into a model or, better yet, a swan. Now, I wasn't looking to be a model but I was not quite expecting what I got either. Have you ever seen that movie *Nightmare Before Christmas*? I was feeling and looking more like Sally. I was a patchwork rag doll with a mass of stitches and scars. But then again, it was great to have cleavage again, to be able to wear a shirt and not worry that if I bent over too much, that someone would see my missing breast. Hey, is that possible? SEE my MISSING breast.

Anyway, my hairstyle was also not helping matters. I was looking a lot like the bad guy, Syndrome, from the movie *The Incredibles*, with the hair straight up, but hey, hair is hair. Aside from all that, I was definitely on my way back. The process was just going to take much more time than I had originally hoped. And I most certainly did not want to turn into that kid that sits in the back seat of the car who keeps saying, "Are we there yet? Are we there yet? Are we there yet?" So, I just did my best to focus on the play and stop bugging God about it.

Believe it or not, I finally got asked out on a date. Might I add, by a handsome, successful, and very easygoing man. I was so thrown off-guard by the invitation that I said yes without thinking. I had had a long-standing business relationship with this man for about eight years, so I told myself that he was just a friend. I instantly felt giddy like a schoolgirl. I must admit, it was a bit silly. I had always found this man to be very good looking with a great personality, which made me feel flattered. The giddiness lasted about a week. I knew that I was still married, and I had made a commitment to myself that I would not date until I was once again single. I wanted to be a woman of integrity. Integrity is something that one must achieve.

My husband had been telling people for a very long time, including my own attorney, that I had gone back to my first husband Paul, which was simply not true. I chose to never try and defend my honor. I would let the truth stand for itself. After the first week of back-and-forth calls, I became very insecure all over again. It was bad; I ran to the mirror, saying, "Oh my God, I can't fix this." The man who asked me out had not seen me in over three years. I looked nothing like I had when I saw him on a regular basis. What if, when he saw me, he wanted out of the date? What if he thought, wow, she sure has aged badly. What if, What if, What if. SSSSSSSSSTOP! If he wanted out when he saw me, then he would be the type of man I should run from anyway. I was doing the same thing I had done all my life. I was looking to be accepted. For days, different scenarios ran through my head. I was obviously not ready for this, plus I did not have my divorce yet. After a few phone calls, I stopped answering the phone and played phone message tag for a while, and then I simply let it die down. It was just not time; I was still a complete mess. But it did give my ego a very much-needed shot in the arm, but when the shot wore off, then the negativity set in; it came on thick.

In one afternoon, I managed to have myself convinced that everyone would be better off if I was not here. My dad was having his own financial setbacks but if I was not here, then maybe he could sell the house I was living in and have a sizable amount in the bank. My kids could just go with their father and let him figure it out for once. My life insurance policy would pay all my bills. The play at the church would go on because, remember, I had all that backup, and I was simply tired. As a person, I could not see a point to my being here. As a person, I was not complete. I kept remembering that movie *Jerry McGuire* when he says at the end, "You complete me." And you know something? I had believed in that "you complete me" theory for so long that I never took the time to become complete in myself. I always thought a man was needed in order for that to happen. I now know that I must first become complete as a woman before I can become complete with man. All it takes is God. I want to become complete through God first and then maybe think about becoming involved later. Once I become complete, only then will I have something solid to offer someone else. Finding someone to complete me and putting that kind of responsibility on someone else is a mistake and unfair.

Although God has graciously given me all these incredible revelations in these pages, I must learn to apply them and live them in order for me to be able to repair my spirit as well as restore my confidence and self-worth.

It is time to open the floodgates of heaven so that we may live a full and abundant life, the full and abundant life that God has promised us. I started to see my old life with Michael as blocked by a series of floodgates that I had put into position in order to protect myself from certain hurts and abuses. I had been living in a survival mode for over twelve years, which also meant that I had shut down my thinking, speaking, feelings, opinions, and even dreaming in a blind, vain attempt to hang on until I could find my footing or some glimmer of hope again. I recently came to realize that all the things I had done to protect myself actually ended up blocking myself off from any help getting through. Much like a floodgate holds back water, I had shut myself off from any and all help. It wasn't until my abuser was gone, and I started actually opening up those floodgates, one by one, that my blessings started to get through. I will now work on me, strengthening Deborah. Yes, I have sustained a great deal of damage but the great thing with God is that through God, all things are possible.

This book is a perfect example. I wrote this during the most horrific time in my life, and God turned it into one of my biggest accomplishments to date, after my children, of course.

I wish I could say that I made it through everything, including the divorce and the cancer, with an A+ on my report card, but this is just not the case. It was on a Tuesday that I started to become unraveled. I had no money, had piling bills, was still in recovery mode, and was sick of the things that seemed not to affect Michael. I had no divorce, my income tax refund was taken away again for the third year in a row because of Michael's back taxes, and my hands were completely tied.

I was at work, standing at the counter, when one of my employees nonchalantly said, "Oh hey, your husband came in the store yesterday and showed me the latest project that he produced; dude, I'm impressed." That was all it took to start my meltdown. I just went off on my employee. I said, "Oh yeah?! Is that what impresses you? You know what impresses me, Jerry? Character! You want to be impressed? Try this: How about the time Michael threw me into a wall so hard that I left my impression in the wall to the point that he had to have his dad come the very next day to patch it up? Does that impress you?" I just kept going with all kinds of trash talking. I had had it. I wanted my turn. There is an old *Gumby* episode that came to mind. Do you remember Gumby? He was once a little green slab of clay.... Anyway, in one of the shows, I remember a kid sitting on a planet, evil looking, saying, "Get off of my world," and that is how I felt. Why did this guy have to continuously come into my place of business tooting his own horn, talking his big talk, flashing his money, his new phone, his new projects? I mean, come on, get a clue. Go to another store for your needs. What? The rest of the world isn't big enough for you? This went on for three days.

Everything seemed astronomically unfair as well as unjust. Maybe God had just said "no" to me. You know that "no" is sometimes God's answer. Maybe I just had it wrong for the umpteenth time. Have you ever heard of that saying, "always a day late and a dollar short"? I found out on the third day of my meltdown that my divorce was finalized on the day I started this tantrum. What were the odds? I was disappointed in my behavior but absolutely in awe that it was over. That was the last floodgate that needed to be dealt with and released. I was in shock; I did not even get it at first when my lawyer called; she said, "Hello, may I please speak to Ms. Deborah Cosio?" I laughed and cried for hours with joy and elation. It felt like a weight had been lifted. You know that heavy lead thing that they lay over you at the dentist office to protect your body during an x-ray? It felt like that had been lifted off of my body; I had a physical experience. I had to be sensitive to my girls. I was not sure how they were going to take it. So I held off on my personal parade.

My son came home with a couple of friends, and when I told them why I was freaking, they joined in the celebration. As the news slowly spread, people were just plain happy for me. It was over. Everything seemed bright. Even taking a deep breath came easier. I could start again.

35

It Is Time to Spread
My Newfound Wings

The wholeness of who you are should not depend on another person. It should not hinge on your spouse, children, parents, or friends. If who you are is dependent on someone else, then what you end up doing is shifting the responsibility of you onto someone else, and in doing that, there is no guarantee of who "you" will end up being. As you can see, my disorder began at a very early age. Unfortunately, as an adult, I ran into a person who was abusive and capitalized on my weakness of needing to be loved, making Adam's Rib Disorder mine to contend with. If we can learn to recognize the early stages of ARD, we can stop a lot of unnecessary pain and heartache.

This warning is not just for the abused but also for the witness of abuse. To you I say, where there is smoke, there is fire (or at least soon will be). Be aware of the possibilities that surround you. I was far from being streetwise and was completely unaware of what was happening to me at the hands of my second husband. Had I been educated in this condition, or if I had even heard about it, I would have had a chance to protect and defend myself.

So, here we are in the last chapter, and I now understand. We were not created to be abused by anyone. I will not embrace cruel, mean, hurtful people in my life or in the lives of my children ever again. I stand before you, complete within myself, through God. I will now protect as well as defend who I am and my destiny from being destroyed. This book is my first step in my endeavor to educate the public to recognize Adam's Rib Disorder. There is no excuse for abuse.

I remember the first song I heard when I got in the car after finding out that my divorce was final. It was a Christina Aguilera song entitled *Soar*. It had such new meaning. I was in the car by myself, singing at the top of my lungs, with tears and all. It was my victory song. I felt as if Christina, who wrote the song, somehow knew me. We had been in the same place. Not only had we been in the same place but we also figured out how to overcome as well. Spread your wings and soar.

SOAR
BY CHRISTINA AGUILERA

It's in your hands. The world is yours.
Don't hold back and always know, all the answers will unfold
What are you waiting for, spread your wings and soar.

In order for you to get God on a deeper level, does it mean you have to go through a horrid divorce? No, that just happens to be where I was when I decided to dig in. Do you have to get breast cancer? No, that just happens to be where I was when I decided to not be moved. It does not matter where you are in life. God is ready. He has always been ready. He is waiting on you. As in any close relationship, it will take a lot of time and effort on your part. You would be surprised how many blessings you miss in the form of people. Michael had no idea what he had in me as a friend, or should I say, what he lost in losing me in his life, just as I had no idea what I was losing when I walked out on my first husband.

Make no mistake. God does not bring the abuse into our lives. We are responsible for the abuse we choose to embrace. In the same respect, we are responsible for the abuse we choose to say "no more" to as well. It is time to open the floodgates so that you may live a full and abundant life, the life that God has promised us. In the seventies, there was a song by Helen Reddy which became very popular entitled I Am Woman. It became a popular theme for many women to live by and I used to live my life saying, "I am woman, hear me roar," but now that I have looked death straight in the face and was able to walk away, I live my life singing, "I am woman, watch me soar."

THE END
OR SHOULD I SAY,
THE BEGINNING

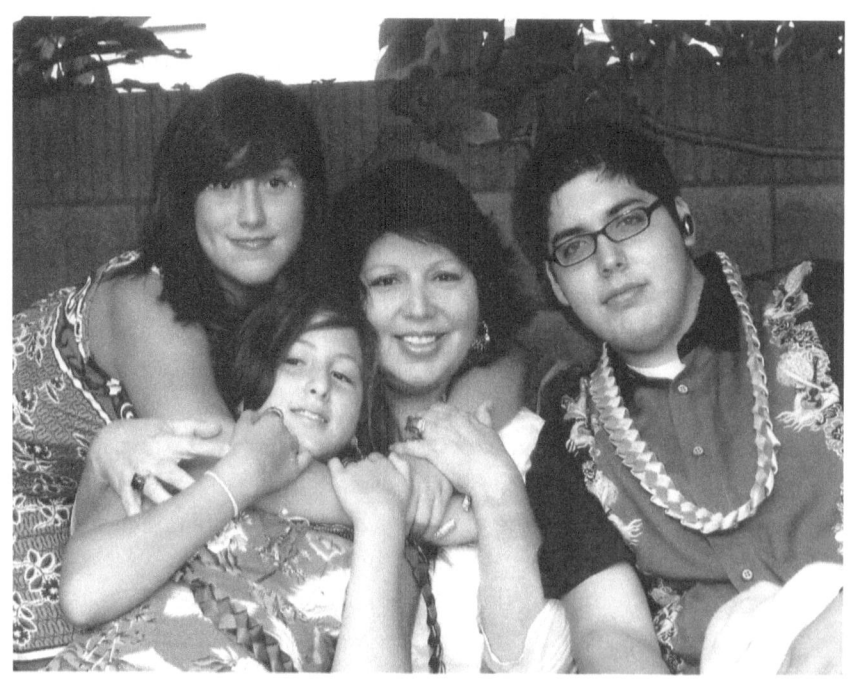

Prayer of Salvation

If you find that you are ready to give your life to Jesus, start with this prayer of salvation. If you are re-dedicating your life to Jesus start new and fresh with this prayer as well.

Father, I know that I am a sinner. I ask that you forgive me of all my sins. I believe that Jesus died on the cross for me. I believe that He was buried and rose on the third day. I now ask you to come into my heart as my Lord and Savior and change my life. Help me to serve you and embrace your characteristics'. I choose to abandon my will and I pray for your will in my life. In Jesus mighty name I pray. Amen

Please know that if you prayed that prayer that is only the beginning. God will do his part but you will also need to do your part. Get into church, pray, worship, read and what ever else it take for you to get closer to God. The more you put in the deeper your relationship with God will become. Remember that no man will ever be able to love you more than God.

www.ingramcontent.com/pod-product-compliance
Lightning Source LLC
Chambersburg PA
CBHW020913290526

45784CB00002BA/534